Challenges in Counselling: Self-Harm

Andrew Reeves

Orders: please contact Bookpoint Ltd, 130 Milton Park, Abingdon, Oxon OX14 4SB. Telephone: (44) 01235 827720. Fax: (44) 01235 400454. Lines are open from 9.00 - 5.00, Monday to Saturday, with a 24 hour message answering service. You can also order through our website www.hoddereducation.co.uk

If you have any comments to make about this, or any of our other titles, please send them to educationenquiries@hodder.co.uk

British Library Cataloguing in Publication Data

A catalogue record for this title is available from the British Library

ISBN: 978 1 444 1 8766 3

Published 2013

Impression number   10 9 8 7 6 5 4 3 2 1

Year   2016 2015 2014 2013

Illustrations by Ian McMillan

Cover photo © Richard Johnson/iStockphoto.com. Photograph posed by a model.

Typeset by Datapage (India) Pvt. Ltd.

Printed and bound by CPI Group (UK) Ltd., Croydon, CR0 4YY for Hodder Education, an Hachette UK Company, 338 Euston Road, London, NW1 3BH.

Contents

Foreword

When I was asked to contribute a book for this new series on working with self-harm it quickly became apparent to me that there were a number of important messages I wanted to convey. First, I wanted to challenge what I consider to be a pervasive and unhelpful position taken in much of the writing of a demarcation between a 'them and us': there are those people who self-harm, and the rest of us who do not. It is my assertion throughout this book that we all have patterns of behaviours in response to stress or difficulty that have the potential to be self-harmful. For me there is no 'them and us', just 'us'. In taking this position I think that we can better connect in counselling with people where self-harm is part of the narrative. Second, to highlight the pull we can often experience in counselling to become self-harm focused, rather than remaining client-centred (in the widest sense of the phrase). Sometimes clients will want to focus on their self-harm, but often they won't. Instead, self-harm as a symptom of hurt will best be addressed through the exploration and resolution of that hurt.

Finally, the importance of self-care. This is an ethical requirement for good practice and something we will quickly say we subscribe to, but something that can easily become peripheral in the face of the day-to-day demands of practice. The irony is that we all too easily neglect self-care, and yet still encourage it in others. This brings us back to point one: if we neglect self-care in working with self-harm, perhaps we are closer to self-harm than we imagined. However, my aim is not to preach a position, but hopefully to offer a book that raises questions and explores areas that will be of help to you in your work with clients. Do feel free to dip in to different sections as and when they are helpful to you; I hope you will find something of a resource for you and your work.

There are a number of people who I would like to thank for their help in the preparation and writing of this book. Kirsten Amis, as Series Editor, has been a constant source of support, encouragement, witty feedback and occasionally very funny emails. Certainly I would not have written this book without her invitation and inspiration. Ian Macmillan, who provided fantastic illustrations to breathe further life into the writing, managing to do so with care and sensitivity. All the editorial and production staff at Hodder Education for their professional management of the text from its early beginnings through to print.

Finally, and not least, to Diane, Adam, Katie and Emily; they are always there, willing to share in the lows and highs of moving from a blank page to a finished book.

Andrew Reeves
Liverpool, 2013

Chapter 1
Introduction and context

The purpose of this series of books is to consider, in some depth, challenges that counsellors face when working with clients. There is no doubt that the therapeutic **process**, from the initial contact with a new client, through to a satisfactory end-point where the client is able to leave therapy having achieved their goals, can be a profound experience for both counsellor and client alike. Of course, many therapeutic relationships will find their own direction, and often (and frustratingly for many trainees) definable 'beginnings', 'middles' and 'ends' are not apparent without the benefit of hindsight. Whatever the nature and course of therapy with a client, there will undoubtedly be challenges to respond to, either for the counsellor to manage or, more commonly, through negotiation with their client.

Clients will present with their own unique **narrative** that gives account of **inter-** and **intra-personal** distress that can, at times, be overwhelming for them. Even if we consider particular 'types' of narratives – or **meta-narratives** – such as depression, anxiety or loss for example, the specific aspects that are unique to that particular client will outweigh those that might be generalised to any type of meta-narrative. That is to say, while we might share common experiences as a consequence of our distress, (for example, loss of appetite, poor sleep patterns, social withdrawal that might accompany a meta-narrative of depression) the uniqueness of our particular experience of a situation will always become paramount. This reality gives rise to a particular challenge, when writing about challenges.

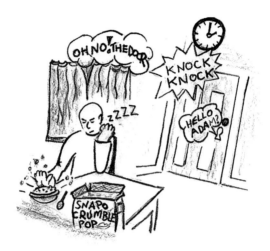

Figure 1.1 Meta-narrative

This particular book in the series is about working with self-harm. Here we immediately fall into an area of difficulty in that 'self-harm' will mean many different things to different people and each individual's experience of self-harm will reflect, in any given moment, their experience of themselves and their world. For counsellors it is likely that the term 'self-harm' will trigger certain responses, thoughts, feelings, assumptions and preconceptions that have the potential to hinder the development of a trusting therapeutic relationship, rather than facilitate it. Here we have two intra-personal processes that need to find a meeting point: a space where one can truly meet the 'other'.

The aim of this particular chapter therefore, is to set a context in which we can begin to consider self-harm and have a shared language, at least temporarily, through which we can explore the dynamics of self-harm and reflect on how we, as counsellors, might successfully negotiate for ourselves and with our clients any challenges that emerge. I therefore propose to consider the following aspects in setting that context:

- definitions: what exactly do we mean by 'self-harm'?
- philosophical positions regarding self-harm
- the nature and extent of self-harm in the UK
- the challenge of working with risk – what we think we should do.

Definitions: what exactly do we mean by 'self-harm'?

There are a number of definitions available that try to help us understand what is meant by 'self-harm'. What will quickly become apparent, however, is that some definitions include some types of behaviours, while excluding others, and other definitions will include a wider set of behaviours, while further excluding more: some are narrow definitions and some more encompassing, yet there are few definitions that perhaps really capture the essence of what is meant by 'self-harm'.

The National Institute for Health and Clinical Excellence (NICE, 2011, p. 3) in their guidance for longer-term management of self-harm define it as,

> 'any act of self-poisoning or self-injury carried out by an individual irrespective of motivation. This commonly involves self-poisoning with medication or self-injury by cutting. There are several important exclusions that this term is not intended to cover. These include harm to the self arising from excessive consumption of alcohol or recreational drugs, or from starvation arising from anorexia nervosa, or accidental harm to oneself'

In providing this first working definition we come across a mixture of different terms used by people at different times. For the most part terms such as 'self-harm', 'self-injury', 'self-mutilation' or 'self-poisoning' are used interchangeably by people to essentially describe the same thing: self-harm. Some will talk about people who self-injure, while others about people who self-harm, but there will not be any meaningful demarcation between how the terms are used. In the NICE definition, however, the term 'self-poisoning' is specifically meant to describe overdosing medication for example, and self-injury describes behaviours such as cutting. The definition excludes behaviour that falls beyond these specific parameters.

The 2004 NICE definition of self-harm states,

> 'self-poisoning or injury, irrespective of the apparent purpose of the act. Self-harm is an expression of personal distress, not an

illness, and there are many varied reasons for a person to harm him or herself'

(NICE, 2004, p. 7)

Again, the same specific nature of the definition can be seen in terms of self-injury and self-poisoning, but this definition then positions self-harm as an 'expression of personal distress' with 'many varied reasons'. It can be said therefore, that the definition clearly places self-harm as a psychological, rather than medical or psychiatric, process.

The Royal College of Psychiatrists in their report *Self-Harm, Suicide and Risk: Helping People Who Self-Harm* (Royal College of Psychiatrists, 2010, p. 21) state that self-harm includes,

> *'intentional acts of self-poisoning or self-injury irrespective of the type of motivation or degree of suicidal intent... [and] it includes suicide attempts as well as acts where little or no suicidal intent at all is involved, for example when people harm themselves as a form of interpersonal communication of distress or other difficult feelings to reduce internal tension or to punish themselves'*

The important relationship between self-harm and suicide risk is flagged in this particular definition, which I will explore in more detail later in the book.

Babiker and Arnold (1997, p. 2) suggest that self-harm is, 'An act which involves deliberately inflicting pain and/or injury to one's body, but without suicidal intent' (thus contradicting the Royal College of Psychiatrists Report, which included suicidal intent). Pembroke (1996, p. 6) states that self-harm is,

> *'Injury to the self which is sometimes spontaneous and sudden with little awareness or conscious thought. Alternatively, the drive to self harm may be powerfully constant and unrelenting with a conscious battle raging. Self harm is about self worth, self preservation, lack of choices and coping with the uncopable.'*

Perhaps the most powerful and succinct definition was one offered by the National Self-Harm Network on their website (1998), who simply stated that self-harm, 'is frequently the least possible amount of damage and represents extreme self-restraint.'

As may be immediately apparent, the definitions are complex, sometimes convoluted, confusing and occasionally contradictory. If we distill from these definitions those essential components we might determine that self-harm:

- can be direct against the body (for example, cutting, burning), which might be termed self-injury
- can include behaviours without immediate impact, (such as eating disorders, risky sexual behaviour)
- may be planned and form part of an **habitual** pattern, or may be unplanned and spontaneous
- may be about coping, living, surviving, and self-worth
- can have a relationship with suicidal potential.

Self-harm therefore is quite a broad term that might encompass a range of different behaviours and perspectives. Much research into self-harm defines it in quite a narrow way, in that direct self-injury, such as cutting and burning, is the only type of self-harm included for statistical analysis or in treatment guidelines, whereas other publications might consider self-harm as a wider term. For the purposes of this book I will include direct and indirect harm, as well as seeing self-harm as a strategy for coping, as well as one for self-punishment, etc.

Babiker and Arnold (1997, p. 4) organise types of behaviours into different categories of self-harm:

- **Self-injury/mutilation**
  - Cutting
  - Scraping
  - Burning
  - Banging
  - Hair pulling (trichotillomania)
- **Other marginal self-injurious behaviours**
  - Smoking
  - Danger sports
  - Reckless driving
  - Workaholism
  - Over-exercise

- **Self-destructive behaviours**
  - Eating disorders
  - Substance abuse
  - Sexual risk-taking
- **Self-harm**
  - Suicide
  - Parasuicide
  - Overdose
- **Factitious disorders**
  - Munchausen's disorder
  - Simulated illness
- **Somatising disorders**
  - Skin disorders
  - Pain
  - Accident prone-ness
- **Body enhancement**
  - Cosmetic surgery
  - Tattooing
  - Piercing
  - Bleaching

This is an interesting list as it captures a range of behaviours and actions on a continuum, moving from actions that are direct with an immediate consequence (such as cutting), through to indirect behaviours with a deferred consequence (such as workaholism). The direct or indirect nature of the behaviour may be meaningful for the client and we will consider later in the book how that might be explored within a therapeutic frame.

This is not intended to be an exhaustive list, and some of the items listed may well be controversial. For example, we admire and praise those who undertake dangerous sports for their bravery, resilience and determination; why then include in a list about self-harm? I will explore throughout the book that an important aspect of working with self-harm is connecting with the meaning of the behaviour, rather than focusing necessarily on the behaviour itself. It is for this reason that I do not intend to spend a great deal of time working through each behaviour, but rather look at what different behaviours might mean for different people. In this context we might include a number of activities that, in and of themselves, might not usually be associated with self-harm.

The nature and extent of self-harm in the UK

It is notoriously difficult to provide any definite or absolutely reliable statistics that accurately reflect the extent of self-harm in the UK. There are a number of reasons for this, including: the differences in definitions of self-harm; a lack of consistency of what is meant by self-harm; no clear central point for collecting such data; the range of agencies and professionals that self-harm might present to; and that much self-harm never actually comes to the attention of agencies or professionals – instead being managed by individuals themselves, often in private. It is this latter point that perhaps make statistics around self-harm so unreliable. From my own experience of working as a counsellor, the overwhelming majority of people I have seen over the years, where self-harm has been a feature of their difficulties, have never spoken to anyone else about it, including family, friends, school, employers – and neither have they attended Accident and Emergency departments (A&E) for help. A great deal of self-harm is invisible to agencies who might record such data and, therefore, statistics for self-harm tend to be **extrapolated** from smaller data sets. That is to say, educated guesses are made about numbers in a wider population from figures derived from smaller populations.

Horrocks *et al.* (2002) suggest that across Europe, the UK has one of the highest rates of self-harm at around 400 people per 100,000. Kapur *et al* (1998) estimated there were approximately 170,000 admissions to A&E departments each year in England. Melzer *et al.* (2002) suggest that, in the UK, between 4.6 per cent and 6.6 per cent of the population have self-harmed. According to the Mental Health Foundation (2006) the average age for the onset of self-harm is 12 years old, while it is estimated that 25,000 young people are seen in A&E departments each year in the UK. Extrapolated figures suggest that 1 million adolescents have considered self-harm, while 800,000 have actually inflicted injuries on themselves (Mental Health Foundation, 2006).

These figures must be read in the context of difficulties in collating accurate figures for self-harm, as outlined previously. However, they do indicate the extent of the issue and the likelihood of self-harm being present in a therapeutic process, either as a specific issue for clients to attend to, or as part of a wider struggle with distress.

A philosophical position regarding self-harm

Having outlined a number of definitions of self-harm and considered the different types of behaviours that might constitute self-harm, it is important for me to outline a philosophical position in writing this book. This position will inform all of the content and discussion that I will offer and is therefore worth stating, and deconstructing, a little. In this regard I bring my own perspective both to my writing, and to how I might approach working with self-harm in counselling. However, throughout the book I will endeavour, wherever possible, to describe key differences in how counsellors from different modalities might approach such work. For example, a person-centred counsellor might conceptualise, and thus work, quite differently with someone who self-harms than perhaps a psychodynamic or cognitive-behavioural counsellor. I will consider these differences through the use of case studies and examples from practice. There will also be important similarities across modalities and I will flag these too.

What is apparent in the definitions of self-harm offered above is how they all generally categorise self-harm as a distinct behaviour undertaken by a specific, and thus defined, group of people. This position permeates a great deal of the literature on self-harm: that is, there are people who self-harm and there are people who don't. This position has validity when considered within the context of particular types of behaviours, but when we think about self-harm at a **process** level, the distinction becomes a little more blurred. For example, consider the five case vignettes here.

Voices

Judie

Judie is a 14-year-old young woman who has experienced bullying at school. She does not feel that she 'fits in', nor that anyone really understands her. She therefore feels quite disconnected from others, and herself. She read a fiction book in which the main character used to cut herself with a razor blade, describing how the character would feel a mixture of relief and a sense of self-validation on seeing her own blood. In identifying with the main character Judie began to cut herself with a razor blade, experiencing similar sorts of feelings. She now cuts herself on her upper arms and upper legs two or three times per week, and has done so for several months.

Voices

Kathy

Kathy began to self-harm when she was a late teenager, and she is now 29 years old. Initially she used to scratch herself, but quickly changed her behaviour and began to pull her hair. She would 'pluck' her eyebrows with her fingers, and then began to pull individual strands of hair out of her head. This developed and, at the worst times, Kathy would pull out larger clumps of hair leaving bald patches, which she would disguise by wearing hats and scarves. Over recent years Kathy has managed to stop excessive hair pulling, but still regularly plucks her eyebrows with her fingers.

Voices

Tosh

Tosh is 17 years old and has always felt a bit 'rubbish' about himself, comparing himself negatively to his friends. Particularly, he feels badly about his body: he believes he is 'thin, weedy and pathetic'. On the other hand he sees all his male friends as stronger, fitter and with better bodies. Tosh has been a member of a gym for several months but has not seen the physical gains he had hoped for. He bought some steroids and has been taking these for a few weeks. He goes to the gym five or six days per week and undertakes a weights routine for several hours at a time. He is feeling exhausted a great deal of the time with little energy for his studies, family or friends.

Voices

Michael

When Michael was 15 years old he began to take recreational drugs and started drinking heavily with friends. This quickly developed into a weekly routine, causing other problems in his life, including relationship difficulties with his family. Michael began to feel that his life was chaotic and he spent a great deal of time feeling angry. He started to initiate fights when he was on a night out. He was often injured during these exchanges but Michael said he felt 'nothing' in response to either what was happening generally, or the injuries he was suffering.

Voices

Weston

Weston is a 36-year-old counsellor. He works in a health care setting and sees six or sometimes seven clients a day, five days per week. At the weekend he has a private counselling practice where he sees an additional five or six clients over the weekend. He has a young family with his partner but usually feels too exhausted to spend any time with them. He feels a financial burden, but also believes that it is essential he builds up experience as a counsellor to help him further his career and create job opportunities for himself in the future.

Activity

Think about the five case vignettes and reflect on the following questions:

1 In relation to Babiker and Arnold's categorisation of self-harming behaviour, in which group would you classify each behaviour?
2 Does it help, or not, to classify the behaviours in this way? Why?
3 Would you consider all the case vignettes to represent self-harm?
4 Which ones would you consider to be 'direct' self-harm, and which 'indirect' self-harm?
5 From your perspective, which ones are more 'serious', and why?
6 How might you explain each case vignette in terms of the behaviour of the person, and the process that might underpin the behaviour?

As we can see from these five case vignettes, we may relate to some, but not to others. We might consider that Judie self-harms because she cuts herself and see a distinction between Judie's behaviour and our own, if we do not cut ourselves. However, we might think a little about Weston's workaholism and, while it may be a little extreme, recognise some aspects of his behaviour in our own. At a behavioural level we can make such distinctions. However, if we revisit the case vignettes from a process perspective, that is, what each person might be feeling 'underneath' the behaviour, more similarities than differences begin to emerge. For instance, if we think about what each person might be feeling we could identify, for example:

● shame
● embarrassment
● low self-esteem
● self-disregard

- fear
- loathing
- punishment.

These feelings, and others, might be apparent across all case vignettes. What is common across all vignettes is a level of dissociation, that is, a level of disconnection between feeling and experience of feeling. All these people are struggling with the types of feelings listed above, but finding safe, meaningful and appropriate ways of expressing these feelings is harder than dissociation. As such, feelings can be expressed through what we do and, if what we feel is difficult or upsetting, what we do can become self-harmful. At this process level of understanding and defining self-harm we can begin to identify thoughts, feelings and behaviours that might not necessarily be that much different from our own. From this perspective therefore, we can begin to challenge the idea that there are people who self-harm, and there are people who do not. It is my intention throughout this book to work from an assumption that, in some way, we ALL self-harm: there is no 'them and us'.

This is an important, and perhaps contentious, philosophical position to take. Important because it provides us with opportunities to begin to reflect on our own self-harming processes: how we feel, how we do not feel, and things we might do as a means of coping with difficult feelings or stresses. Contentious because most literature on self-harm differentiates between those who 'do', and 'us'. It is an unhelpful and, as I have argued here, false demarcation in that we can all do things as a means of coping that might be harmful to ourselves, rather than expressing our true feelings. Think of the times when you have worked too hard, or gone into work feeling unwell. Or perhaps had too much drink as a means of dealing with stresses. Or instead done something in frustration that hurt yourself physically, rather than paying attention to your needs? There is clearly a difference between these examples and cutting ourselves in the depths of despair, but, at a process level, the more we understand about our own ways of dealing (or not dealing) with difficult things, the more insight, understanding, compassion and empathy we might achieve with our clients.

The challenge of working with risk – what we think we should do

I will explore things we might need to do in response to self-harm that has the potential to put a client at risk to themselves (or others) in later chapters, including those related to professional issues (Chapter 7) and ethical issues (Chapter 8). Additionally, our concerns and fears about clients at risk are also important in how they shape our anxieties about self-harm, which again we will explore in more detail later. I briefly wanted to outline the issues of self- and professional expectations about working with risk in this introductory chapter because I believe it is so fundamentally important in shaping, and sometimes gets in the way of, the therapeutic process.

The literature suggests an important link between self-harm and suicide potential (Owens et al, 2002; Hawton et al, 2003; Winter et al, 2012a; 2012b). As counsellors we will typically contract with our clients an agreement of confidentiality that is, in part, boundaried by risk to self or others. I will talk later about the fears of 'getting it wrong' with suicidal clients, but it is in this context that we might fear working with people who self-harm; that they may kill themselves and that we might have a duty to prevent them from doing so. It is a complex area that requires commensurate attention, but one we can also stumble over with insufficient thought.

It is important to remember that statistical links, while important, do not necessarily always translate to the realities of the therapeutic relationship we encounter: one event does not necessarily lead to another. For example, in relation to suicide, Schneidman (1996) asks us to reflect on the fact that many people who talk about suicide do not make an attempt on their own life, yet many people who die through suicide have talked about the possibility. From this challenge we can see the conundrum: given that most people who die through suicide will have talked to someone about the possibility of suicide we might be lead to assume that most people who talk about suicide will act on their thoughts, yet this is not the case. Likewise, that many people who die through suicide might have a history of self-harm does not necessarily mean that most people who self-harm will go on to end their lives through suicide. It is a statistical anomaly that challenges our anxiety in how best to respond to risk. My intention here is not to diminish the potential risk, nor suggest that self-harm should not be carefully considered with clients in counselling, but rather to challenge any presumption that one automatically equates to the other.

Summary

As I have outlined in this introductory chapter, self-harm is notoriously difficult to define with any clarity beyond specific behaviours, such as cutting. Statistics for self-harm are notoriously inaccurate given difficulties in collecting such data and that much self-harm is managed by the individuals themselves, never coming to the attention of agencies, professionals, families or friends. In that context, however, the likelihood of counsellors working with clients who self-harm is extremely high and therefore the challenge is for counsellors to carefully reflect on their understanding of self-harm, how they conceptualise it, and how they respond to it in a wider phenomenological sense (thoughts, feelings, reactions and responses, for example). In doing this counsellors can helpfully reflect on their own processes that might speak something of self-harm as a means of engendering empathy and psychological contact with clients to help them explore often difficult and otherwise inaccessible areas of their lives.

Further reading

Babiker, G. & Arnold, L. (1997) *The Language of Injury: Comprehending Self-Mutilation*. Oxford: Wiley-Blackwell.

National Self-Harm Network (1998) *Self-injury: myths and common sense*. National Self-Harm Network. **www.nshn.co.uk/facts.html**

Chapter 2
Settings

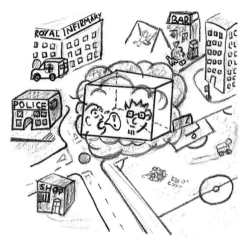

Figure 2.1 Counselling never takes place in a vacuum

Counselling in Context

There is always a context for counselling. That is, counselling never takes place in a vacuum, disconnected from any other system or influence. As counsellors therefore, we need to pay careful attention to that context and consider how it influences and shapes the nature and form of the therapeutic **process** and relationship, because it certainly will. While this may appear an obvious statement to make, it is not uncommon for counsellors to engage in their work with clients and become so immersed in the intricacies of that work they forget what sits beyond the door. Often I have become so captured by a client's **narrative**, or the process of the relationship, that I have overlooked important factors and information that might further inform or shape the work. Certainly in my own counsellor training, many years ago, the primary focus was on the nature of the relationship, with less time being spent exploring those aspects that might be integral to that relationship, other than the most apparent ones, such as ethics.

The context of counselling therefore, comes in all sorts of shapes and sizes and I would group them into: relational; ethics and values; law; policy and procedural; and organisational.

Relational factors
- The client's personal and family history
- The counsellor's personal and family history
- The nature of previous relationships for both counsellor and client
- Expectations and goals for counselling, either explicitly stated or implicitly held
- **Transferential** or **countertransferential** dynamics

Ethical and value-based factors
- The ethical framework in which the counsellor works, if any, (BACP, UKCP, BABCP, etc.)
- The ethical framework of the organisation in which counselling takes place
- The training of the counsellor
- The **modality** being practiced
- The **world-view** of the client
- The world-view of the counsellor

Legal factors
- General legal requirements informing counselling (such as confidentiality; **capacity**; anti-terrorism legislation)
- Specific legal requirements informing counselling particular to an agency (such as adoption; counselling prior to a termination of pregnancy)

Policy and procedural factors
- Working policies informing particular aspects of practice (for example, assessment; working with risk)
- Procedural documents requiring certain courses of action by the counsellor (for example, referral on to another agency in specific situations; working with risk)
- Any overarching procedures pertinent to the organisation in which counselling is located (such as data protection; access to notes)

Organisational factors
- The culture and ethos of the setting in which counselling is located, (for example, **statutory**, such as health or social care, education, etc.)

- Whether the organisation targets its services to particular populations, (for example, young people; older people, etc.)
- The particular view the organisation has about the role and nature of counselling, (such as workplace counselling aimed at reducing levels of staff sickness)

We can see that the list above is also incomplete, and that other factors might also be added to the many aspects that inform the counselling we offer. In turn, many of these factors will have specific relevance for how we work with clients where self-harm is evident or suspected. The purpose of this chapter is to consider the particular implications of working with clients who self-harm that might arise from specific settings or organisational contexts.

Organisational settings relevant to counselling

It would be a lengthy process to take each of the points above and address each of them fully – particular aspects of them will be considered in more depth in other chapters (such as ethics). I will structure the chapter so that we consider primary aspects as shaped by organisational context: statutory; education; the 'third sector' (voluntary organisations); workplace and employment; and independent practice. In a more general sense we can draw on other disciplines, such as economics, to categorise the types of organisations. Fellman et al (2007) outline five primary categories of systems in society:

1. primary: the production and harvesting of food and goods from the earth (grain, coal, etc.)
2. secondary: the manufacturing of goods (textiles, chemicals, etc.)
3. tertiary: the service industries (health care, law, etc.)
4. quaternary: intellectual industries (government, research, etc.)
5. quinary: the highest level of decision making in society (for example, in government and health care).

I have suggested elsewhere (Reeves, 2013) that counselling is typically delivered at the tertiary level (in health and social care, for example), is informed at the quaternary level (through counselling research) and is structured at a quinary level (through professional organisations). We will focus our discussion at the tertiary level as that is where counselling is actually provided and where the work with self-harm will be primarily experienced. It is worth noting, however, that our work with self-harm will be informed by research, which we will discuss later in the chapter on research (Chapter 9), and also through ethical frameworks outlined by counselling decision-making bodies. For clarification, Fellman talked of the quinary level in a much broader way that I am using it here, locating the categories at a societal level. In this context I am applying the categories to counselling as a structure within its own right.

It is worth taking the headings of organisational contexts outlined previously and defining them a little more clearly. I have previously offered definitions for these organisations (Reeves, 2013, pp. 117–22) and will present them here.

Statutory settings

By statutory settings I refer to centrally funded health and social care organisations, such as the National Health Service (NHS) and social services departments. It is often the case that such organisations have particular statutory responsibilities, as outlined in law, such as child protection and mental health, for example. Counselling can be found in a variety of different contexts within the statutory sector (Reeves, 2013, p. 117):

- primary (general) care (in General Practice settings), including specialist services located within primary care (such as well-women/men services)
- secondary (specialist) care, including:
  - in- and out-patient mental health services
  - cardiovascular units
  - spinal injury units
  - fertility and maternity units
  - head injury units
  - child and adolescent services
  - pain management units
  - services for older people
  - hospices
  - learning disability units
- Improving Access to Psychological Therapies (IAPT) services for adults and children/young people – a government-funded initiative for the treatment of depression and anxiety delivering approved psychological therapies at 'low intensity' (guided self-help; **bibliotherapy**) and 'high intensity' (therapist-delivered interventions) levels.

Social services departments assess social need and deliver social care. Counselling and psychotherapy services may be found in:

- adult services, including:
  - mental health
  - learning difficulties
  - physical impairment
  - older people's services
  - generic 'intake' or 'one-stop shop' centres;
- children and family services, including:
  - child protection
  - family support
  - children's centres
  - family therapy services
  - child and adolescent units
  - sexual abuse support units.

Education settings

Counselling in education settings has a long established tradition and was perhaps embedded in such settings in an organised way prior to it becoming mainstream in health and social care settings. We might initially think of education as being the domain of younger people of school age, but education settings also include further and higher education, which draw from the widest population base in terms of age. While in the UK there may be slight differences between age delineation in England, Scotland, Wales and Northern Ireland, in general terms education settings in which counselling can be found are (Reeves, 2013, p. 118):

- primary education: typically from the ages of 5 years through to 11 years
- secondary education: typically from the ages of 11 years through to 16 years
- further education: typically from 16 years.
- higher education: study for 18-year-olds onwards

The third sector (voluntary organisations)

Third sector organisations fall outside of primary central government funding, although may receive some funding through charitable channels. Instead, they are often registered as charities with specific aims of social benefit, either generally or for specific groups or causes. Many such organisations will employ paid staff to undertake key organisational and structural tasks, but will then rely on a larger number of volunteer workers for the delivery of the 'service'. In this context many counsellors will work for third sector organisations voluntarily.

Third sector organisations offer a very wide range of services in society, including:

- for children and young people
- for young adults
- for people with particular problems or difficulties, (such as drug and alcohol abuse, bereavement)
- for people with eating disorders
- for particularly vulnerable groups, such as suicidal people
- for people with mental health distress
- for people with learning disabilities or physical impairment
- for people within a particular cultural or **demographic** group, (e.g., Asian women, young males).

Each organisation will determine the type and nature of counselling on offer and will develop their own policies and procedures related to the delivery of counselling. So, even though a counsellor may work in a voluntary capacity within a third sector organisation, they will still be required to adhere to the policies and procedures of the organisation.

Workplace and employment counselling

Many larger organisations offer counselling to employees to help attend to welfare considerations. While such counselling may be centred around the well-being of the employee, it is important to note that such counselling is also to facilitate a healthy workforce so that business targets can be met. It is in every company's interests to reduce sickness levels amongst staff and to ensure that employees are best placed to deliver the product or service.

How counselling is offered will be informed by the size of the organisa-tion, the financial resources available to offer counselling and the phi-losophy of the organisation. For example, some large companies employ their own counsellors and therefore keep counselling 'in-house', whereas others will opt to 'buy in' counselling – usually through an Employee Assisted Programme (EAP) – to manage its delivery. An EAP, and there are several in operation in the UK, employs counsellors on a sessional basis and is contracted by the company to manage all aspects of the delivery of counselling. As such, the counsellor might not have direct contact with the employer, rather liaising with the client directly and the link person in the EAP. There is a strong evidence-base for the value and efficacy of workplace counselling (McLeod, 2010).

The independent sector

Counsellors who work independently do so separately from an employing organisation; they are self-employed for the purposes of the delivery of counselling, charging clients directly usually on an hourly basis. Such counsellors will develop and maintain what is usually termed 'a private practice' where they will advertise their services, manage their own referrals, be responsible for the physical location of counselling and, in every other way, take actions to ensure the delivery of an ethical and appropriate counselling provision. I include independent practice here in a chapter looking at organisational settings because independent practice can be seen as a setting within its own right. While the counsellor works independently from employing organisations, the same level of consideration is required to ensure that factors that influence the counselling relationship are fully attended to and followed. For example, an independent counsellor still has the same requirement to work within the law, to follow ethical requirements (if they are a member of a professional organisation that sets such requirements) and to meet their duty of care to the client. They may be independently employed, but are not above the law, ethics and other expectations of good practice. Indeed, many independent practitioners will take steps to develop their own working policies and procedures to ensure all clients are responded to equitably and fairly.

Working with self-harm in organisational contexts

It is important to understand clearly the diversity of settings in which counselling is delivered to begin to contextualise how those settings might inform the nature of work with clients who self-harm. In therapeutic terms it might be argued that there are few qualitative differences in therapy with clients who self-harm across settings and that, more relevantly, the main differences will instead be seen across **modality** and core training. However, while this is true at a **relational** level, there may be important influences that shape the wider approach to self-harm, or how self-harm is understood, based on organisational difference.

Different settings will bring particular perspectives on how such work should take place (or whether people who self-harm should be seen for counselling at all), and will therefore exert influence on counsellors. It is, therefore, worth considering these in turn. It should be noted, however, that the differences between organisational settings as outlined here are not necessarily as clear as they might seem. For example, while perspectives at play in health care settings may differ greatly from those seen in the third sector, there will be health care organisations that adopt approaches more typically found in third sector settings, and vice versa. Positions in relation to self-harm will be informed not only by organisational dynamics, they will also be informed by those who commission, manage and audit services. Whether we consider these factors from a **macro** perspective (at an organisational level), or a **micro** perspective (at an individual level), both will always shape and inform the nature of our work.

It is important to note that across all settings outlined in this chapter, in the UK there is no statutory responsibility for counsellors to break confidentiality with clients who self-harm. Few counsellors would argue with the requirement to pass on child protection concerns, but might not feel so clearly about self-harm. There are inevitably value judgements that are made around confidentiality that occur at an individual and organisational level. It is important to keep this point in mind when thinking about work with self-harm in different contexts: the requirement is not to break confidentiality, but the organisational judgement will change according to setting.

Working with self-harm in the statutory sector

Most organisations might be described as 'risk averse', in that their intention is to deliver services that meet clear parameters around safety and risk. In doing so, it is not untypical for organisations to develop policies and procedures that direct counsellors to act in certain ways when working with clients at risk, including that of self-harm. For many organisations self-harm is strongly associated with suicide potential (as some of the literature affirms, although keeping in mind the caveats outlined in Chapter 1) and, as such, great care is taken to ensure that such clients are assessed appropriately and are able to function within the parameters of the service. This is perhaps particularly true in statutory settings, such as health and social care, where the sense of responsibility is enhanced through the statutory footing of the organisation. Of course, as we have already identified, there is no such thing as a typical health or social care setting, with the provision of services falling across a wide **demographic** and problem focus.

Whilst it is, therefore, difficult to make generalisations, it may be fair to assert that counsellors working in the statutory sector typically do so within clearly defined policies and procedures that require them to act in the event of risk by referring on for consultation or further assessment. The age or perceived level of vulnerability of the client will be an important factor in determining how prescriptive such policies might be.

Clients may be referred to health or social care agencies because of their self-harm, perhaps for further specialist assessment, or as a consequence of a **safeguarding** intervention; or self-harm may become apparent during assessment or in the process of counselling. Consider the following two short client scenarios.

Voices

Tantse

Tantse is 13 years old and has been attending counselling in a Child and Adolescent Mental Health Service (CAMHS) following a GP referral for severe depression. Counselling began following an assessment by the team's psychiatrist and Ged, the counsellor, has been seeing Tantse for several weeks. Tantse discloses during one of the sessions that she has been cutting herself on her arms to manage some difficult feelings, although states these are not necessarily serious and she takes care of them herself. The policy of the CAMHS is that all instances of self-harm must be reported to the psychiatrist for further assessment. Ged is aware of this but also knows that Tantse does not want the psychiatrist to be told.

Voices

Frederick

Frederick is 47 years old and has been referred to a counsellor based within a cardiac care setting following a heart attack several months before. During the counselling, which aimed to help Frederick make emotional and psychological adjustments due to his physical ill-health, he discloses that sometimes he gets very angry. He has started to take 'small overdoses' of the medication prescribed for his cardiac condition, or not take it at all. He does this as a means of 'self-punishment'. His counsellor, Annee, is concerned about Frederick's actions in relation to his physical health and she is also aware of a very strict policy within her service of reporting any medical concerns to the responsible medical officer, in this case Frederick's consultant.

Activity

Think about Tantse's and Frederick's scenarios and reflect on the following questions:

1 In what ways do you think the policies the counsellors work within are informed by the setting? Why?
2 Do you respond differently to the scenarios based on the circumstances, such as age of the client? What informs your responses?
3 What would you do if you were Ged, and why?
4 What would you do if you were Annee, and why?

Working with self-harm in education settings

As we have already outlined, education-based counselling covers a full age group, with different perceived responsibilities for each. For example, counselling with a 7 year old in primary education will be very different to counselling with a 22 year old in higher education. The level of capacity and understanding will be profoundly different. While education settings will have statutory obligations to manage the form and nature of education, they are less related to health and social care. However, for those under 18 years of age, education providers are likely to have a safeguarding policy, which attends to the health and social well-being of students, including child protection. It is under such safeguarding policies that education settings are likely to determine policies around self-harm, requiring counsellors to break confidentiality to the school or other appropriate professional bodies, where self-harm is evident. This is likely to be less clear for those receiving counselling in education settings for those over 18 years of age, where boundaries of confidentiality will be defined differently.

The counsellor in an education setting might be seen as having the specialist knowledge and skills to respond to a client who is self-harming. Often counsellors have more experience than other professionals found in such settings, such as teachers, lecturers or other academic support staff, and will be turned to in response to a crisis (it is not untypical for the **disclosure** of self-harm to be viewed as a crisis by the person who has been disclosed to). Consider Askew's and Tosh's short scenarios.

Voices

Askew

Askew is a 12-year-old boy referred to the school counsellor following several outbursts of bad behaviour in class. He has been unresponsive to teaching and pastoral input and his Head of Year, along with his parents, believe counselling could be beneficial. He is indifferent about counselling but is willing to attend. During his first few sessions with his counsellor, Lynn, he talks of stabbing himself with a pencil in his leg when he gets really angry. He has done this for a few months and thinks it is getting worse.

Voices

Tosh

Tosh is a 20-year-old student in a UK university who attends the university counselling service because of depression. During the assessment session Tosh says that he sometimes feels suicidal, although does not intend to take his own life, but thumps walls and sometimes cuts himself when he feels very sad. His counsellor, Gerald, explores this with him. Tosh says this has been going on 'for a while' and it helps him cope.

Activity

Think about Askew's and Tosh's scenarios and reflect on the following questions:
1   What are the main differences, if any, between the issues for the counsellors working with Askew and Tosh?
2   How might each education setting view self-harm differently, and why?
3   What would you do if you were Lynn, and why?
4   What would you do if you were Gerald, and why?

Working with self-harm in third sector settings

Beyond overarching legal and ethical requirements, very few third sector organisations are constituted in the context of statutory responsibilities (although a minority are, such as those providing counselling prior to the termination of a pregnancy, or an adoption). As such, third sector organisations are likely to develop working protocols and policies based on philosophical, rather than legal, positions. Like all settings, counsellors must be clear that they understand the nature of the organisation's position in relation to self-harm, and if they disagree with it, that they either challenge the policy, work within the confines of the policy or, ultimately, that they leave and work elsewhere. One option, which is not ethical, but is one that too many counsellors follow, is to disagree with the policy and thus disregard it, working in the way they prefer. This leaves them in a very vulnerable position should their work come under scrutiny or be subject to a complaint.

There are some third sector organisations that specialise in working with self-harm and clients may refer themselves to such services. However, as in all settings, self-harm can be present for any client, including more generic third sector organisations. The counsellor has to be able to respond appropriately and in line with organisational expectation. It is difficult to represent fully the breadth of services on offer in the third sector in just two case scenarios, but consider Karen's and Esmy's accounts.

Voices

Karen

Karen, who is 32 years old, has referred herself to a local third sector organisation that offers generic free counselling to adults. She suffers from panic attacks and high anxiety, as well as low self-esteem. During counselling with her counsellor, Dan, she talks of pulling her hair out 'in clumps' and hitting herself when in a rage. She has bruising to her face and neck, which she states is self-inflicted. The organisation has a general risk policy which states that clients should be referred to their GP if they present 'a risk to themselves or others'.

Voices

Esmy

Esmy is a 19-year-old woman who attends for counselling in an organisation that offers support to women who have experienced sexual abuse. The organisation has a very clear policy on confidentiality which states that confidentiaity will be maintained even if the client presents an immediate risk. Esmy's counsellor, Caroline, struggles with this policy and is alarmed when Esmy talks of burning herself on her legs, arms and stomach with an iron.

Activity

Think about Karen's and Esmy's accounts and reflect on the following questions:
1 What are your views about each organisation's confidentiality policy?
2 Do you think organisations should be free to set their own policies, or should there be limitations to confidentiality linked with ethical frameworks? Why do you think that?
3 What would you do if you were Dan, and why?
4 What are the issues for Caroline to address?

Working with self-harm in workplace and employment settings

Counselling in workplace settings is partly informed by the nature of the workplace in which counselling is offered. For example, an organisation might expect different responses from a counsellor if working with someone who has an administrative job, as opposed to someone who works in a 'high-risk' environment (such as operating machinery, etc.). Organisations will be very aware of their duty of care both to their employees and also the wider public. If they believe an employee is permanently or temporarily unfit to undertake their duties they have a responsibility to act accordingly, particularly if the implications involve risk to others. Likewise, EAPs often insist on a clear contract of confidentiality boundaried by risk (amongst other things) for: a) the well-being of the client; b) a responsibility to the employing organisation; and c) fear of accusations of negligence in the event of a client death or other crisis. Counsellors who undertake work for EAPs will typically have to agree to a working contract that binds them to work within the procedural parameters the EAP has established. Like all other employing situations, counsellors who work for workplace counselling organisations directly will commit to work within the organisation's policy.

Where self-harm is apparent, it is not uncommon for workplace counselling organisations or EAPs to make a direct referral to a health or social care agency, rather than undertaking the work directly. However, this is not always the case and counsellors in such settings will be required to have the requisite skills and knowledge to respond appropriately when self-harm emerges as part of the therapeutic process. Consider Vee's and Daley's scenarios.

Voices

Vee

Vee, who is 27 years old, works for a large retail company and has had several episodes of sick leave due to anxiety and depression. She is referred to the workplace counsellor, Angie, and finds the counselling helpful. She talks to Angie about her self-harm, cutting her arms and legs, which she has done since she was 17 years old. Vee knows the company has a strict policy of passing on concerns about risk.

Voices

Daley

Daley is a 57-year-old truck driver who has been referred via an EAP for counselling. He has been off sick for a while following the death of his partner. He tells his counsellor, Joy, that he is drinking heavily as a means of coping. He feels ready to return to work but Joy is concerned that Daley's drinking will impair his capacity to drive vehicles. Daley says this is not an issue.

Working with self-harm as an independent practitioner

As I have outlined, an independent practitioner is someone who works independently from an employing organisation, which means they have much more control over how they respond to particular situations. This might include a very clear boundary limited by risk to self, through to maintaining confidentiality in all situations. What is important, as is the case in all the contexts considered here, is that the counsellor (or agency) clearly communicates the policy of the setting to the client so that the client is able to make an informed choice, where possible, about whether to begin counselling and/or the level of self-disclosure. Independent counsellors therefore, need to reflect carefully, and in supervision, about their level of understanding about self-harm and any personal views that might shape or influence how they would respond to clients.

It is not uncommon for clients to approach an independent counsellor, rather than using one in their workplace or seeing their GP, particularly if there are things they wish to explore that they consider to be difficult, such as self-harm. The hope might be that the counsellor can keep information confidential and that no notes are made on health or employment files. It is therefore essential (as is the case in all settings) for counsellors to communicate clearly what they offer in terms of confidentiality, and to ensure that if working with self-harm that they have the support and supervision in place to enable them to do so. Consider Alexis' and Gareth's scenarios.

Voices

Alexis

Alexis is a counsellor with her own private practice. She strongly believes that clients should not hurt themselves and that it is a wrong thing to do. She has been seeing a client, Sushka, for eight months and they have developed a strong therapeutic relationship. Sushka feels very trusting of Alexis. Sushka tells Alexis of her self-harming (hitting and cutting herself) and Alexis feels thrown into a quandary, caught between her relationship with Sushka and her own views about self-harm.

Voices

Gareth

Gareth has been working as an independent practitioner for several years. He has chosen to develop a very inclusive contract of confidentiality, in that he will not disclose concerns regarding self-harm. His client, Jason, is 16 years old and has been ingesting substances for several months (cleaning fluids). Jason says that he fears he is really causing damage to himself but does not really know how to stop. Gareth has little experience of working with self-harm.

Activity

Think about Alexis' and Gareth's scenarios and reflect on the following questions:

1   What are your thoughts about an independent practitioner developing a working procedure based on their own views about something, in this instance self-harm?
2   What are the benefits and challenges of each of the different perspectives on confidentiality in relation to self-harm?
3   What would you do if you were Alexis, and why?
4   What would you do if you were Gareth, and why?

Summary

We have seen throughout this chapter that while the **intrapersonal process** of self-harm might be similar for individuals, the manner in which it is received and thus potentially responded to, can vary greatly depending on the organisational context in which counselling is located. It is therefore important for you to reflect carefully on the context in which you practice and ensure that you are familiar with any expectations the organisation places on you with respect to self-harm. Failure to do so might mean you respond inappropriately to a client's **disclosure** of self-harm, leaving you or the client in a vulnerable position in the event of difficulty.

Further reading

Fellman, J.D., Getis, A. & Getis, J. (2007) *Human Geography: Landscapes of Human Activities.* Maidenhead: McGraw-Hill.

McLeod, J. (2010) 'The effectiveness of workplace counselling: a systematic review', *Counselling and Psychotherapy Research*, 10 (4): 238–48.

Reeves, A. (2013) *An Introduction to Counselling and Psychotherapy: From Theory to Practice.* London: Sage.

Chapter 3
Theory and skills

We considered in the first chapter reasons why people might harm themselves, and later on, in Chapter 6, we will reflect in more detail on self-harm from an 'inside' perspective, that is, the stages a person might go through in the lead up to, and during, self-harm. The purpose of this chapter is to consider theories and skills that we as counsellors might draw on to help us in our work with clients where self-harm is part of the presentation. As must be reiterated here, for many people counselling will not focus on self-harm specifically at all (even though our own anxiety might draw us to it), but will rather explore the source of difficulties and hurt of which self-harm is a symptom. For other clients, even though self-harm may be a symptom of their distress, it becomes sufficiently prominent and concerning to be an issue in and of itself.

Different models of practice will approach work with clients with different ways of viewing distress and, consequently, different ways of helping. We will see in Chapter 9 that there is a strong evidence-base for the efficacy of CBT in working with self-harm, but perhaps less so for some other approaches, such as from a humanistic frame. It is important to stress that a comparative paucity of research on one approach does not mean that approach is not helpful, nor the strength of evidence for another mean the other is. Instead, the evidence-base can simply reflect a research culture within a particular **modality** and the type of evidence it produces, rather than a clear statement as to whether one approach is better than another.

My position in this chapter is that most recognised models have the potential to be helpful to a client who may be self-harming and that I do not intend to privilege one above another. Instead, it is my assertion that there are a number of important *qualities* that need to be present to ensure work around self-harm is safe and has the potential to be effective. These are:

- Any counsellor must be qualified (or in advanced training) and drawing on a core theoretical model (or integration of models).

- Regular supervision must be in place, meeting at least the minimum requirements of supervision set by relevant professional bodies.
- The counsellor must work within the context of a clear ethical framework.
- Any counselling must be carefully contracted, including clearly setting boundaries around time, availability between sessions and confidentiality.
- The counsellor must be a reflective practitioner, with a willingness to identify professional and personal areas for development and to seek resources to support that development, as appropriate.
- The counsellor must be able to engage with a dialogue around risk and be aware of any existing policies and procedures (where they exist) and work within them accordingly.
- The counsellor needs to make themselves aware of issues around self-harm, including: types of self-harm; why people might self-harm; the consequences of self-harm on the client and those around them; and what research tells us about self-harm; and be willing to explore their own strategies for coping under stress, which might include forms of self-harm.
- The counsellor must be willing to communicate clearly with clients about the client's self-harm.
- The counsellor must be aware of the danger of becoming self-harm focused, where this is not the client's wish or goal.
- The counsellor must not judge, but must be empathic, compassionate and understanding, and willing to be congruent (in line with the teachings of their core theoretical framework).

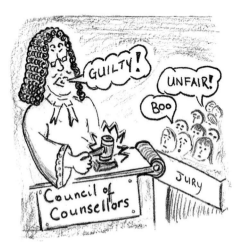

Figure 3.1 The counsellor must not judge

More could probably be added to the list above, but if all these factors are present then it is my assertion that we put ourselves in the best position to offer a safe, respectful and appropriate space for clients to explore their distress. Rather than providing an overview of the four main orientations in counselling (psychodynamic, humanistic, cognitive-behavioural and integrative/pluralistic), which inevitably would be too reductionist to be meaningful, I will instead introduce a client as if they were presenting for counselling and take us through the process of assessment, goal setting and types of interventions that might be helpful. This will also include focusing on a number of key generic counselling skills and how they might be applied to a dialogue with a client about self-harm.

The assumption here is the importance of the relationship between you as counsellor and your client. Fundamentally, it will not matter what skills or interventions you try if the relationship is not in place to create a context for them to be meaningful. As we know, and will discuss further throughout this book, there will be various challenges to the relationship, which must be carefully attended to and negotiated.

Working with self-harm: Zac

The counselling we will consider with Zac, our client, will take place in a generic counselling agency for young people based in the third sector (a voluntary agency for young adults, aged 16–25) which offers free time-limited counselling of up to six sessions. All clients are asked to register by giving contact information, their GP details, their availability and a brief statement about what has brought them to counselling. The demographic information about Zac is:

Age:	18 years
Gender:	Male
Ethnic background:	White European
Disability:	None

On the section of the form where he was asked to provide some detail as to his contact with the agency, he wrote:

'I have been depressed for some time and feel really panicky too on occasions. My GP thought it would be a good idea to come for counselling to try and sort things out. I talk to friends about how I feel but don't want to burden them too much. I sometimes

feel really rough and don't know what to do to help myself. I hope counselling will help me think of different ways of doing this, and to feel better.'

Zac is placed on a waiting list for four weeks and is then given an appointment for an initial session.

The initial session

The session is booked with a counsellor called Louise. Different agencies, counsellors, and ways of working will structure initial sessions quite differently. For example, psychodynamic or CBT work might begin with a comprehensive assessment of Zac's presenting issues, including details of family, history of problems, variations on the severity of problems and Zac's goals for counselling. While other approaches, including some of the humanistic approaches (such as person-centred), might not see the role of assessment as appropriate to the philosophy of their model and would, instead, meet with Zac where he currently is and allow his story to unfold.

However a counsellor decides to approach the initial session, they will be very aware of any factors that might additionally inform the counselling – in this case the fact that counselling is limited to six sessions only. Louise works as an integrative counsellor, drawing on ideas and principles from psychodynamic, humanistic and CBT, but rooting her overall work in a person-centred approach. She undertakes an assessment with all her clients but does so in a dialogic way. That is, she does not use forms or questionnaires but instead has a number of questions to ask Zac that will be prioritised based on what he says. Louise covers a number of areas in her assessment and writes it up – see Box 1.

Box 1: Assessment interview with Zac

Presenting problems

- Zac struggles with depression and has done so for approximately six years (since he was 12 years old)
- Was physically and sexually assaulted by a stranger when he was 11 years old – did not report this to anyone
- He describes low mood (feeling sad, lacking in energy, withdrawn and poor motivation)
- Over recent months he has begun to experience higher levels of anxiety (sweating, awareness of heart rate, panicky, out of breath)
- He feels that he is coping less with his current problems

Functioning and background

- Zac lives alone in rented accommodation
- His parents live close by and he gets on well with both of them, feeling able to talk to them about his problems (particularly his father). He has two siblings, a brother (Jason, aged 22) and a sister (Penny, aged 16) – he describes family relationships as good.
- He works part-time in a shop and is thinking of going to university
- Sleep is poor (difficulties in getting to sleep, or waking early)
- Appetite is generally alright, other than at times of higher anxiety when it is poor
- No current relationship and describes sex drive as low – this has become worse over recent months since anxiety has become more of an issue

Subjective well-being

- Zac has low self-esteem and low self-confidence. He does not believe that many people like him (although has a good network of friends)
- Poor body image – feels he is ugly and does not like his body – too thin
- Is able to talk to friends but is not always sure whether they think he is a nuisance, or a burden to them

Risk

- Zac has occasional suicidal thoughts (of wanting to go to sleep and not wake up), but has no intention of acting on them, nor has a plan
- Describes himself as 'reckless' sometimes, driving quickly without care or picking fights with people
- General lack of self-care
- Zac said there were other things he 'did to cope', but did not wish to elaborate on them

Hopes for counselling

- Zac wants to understand why he feels about himself the way he does
- Would like to learn strategies to manage his anxiety
- Would like to learn ways of supporting himself better

This extensive information came out of dialogue with Zac and provided both Louise and Zac with an important starting point for counselling. For Louise, it gave her an opportunity to understand Zac's struggle in much more detail. For Zac, it was the first time he had talked through everything 'in one go' and he reported finding it extremely helpful in ordering his thoughts about his problems. This is certainly one of the benefits of structured assessment – or structured exploration – early on in counselling. Louise was also able to talk Zac through the policies of the agency, including confidentiality (limited by immediate risk to self and others). Louise believed the underlying factor for Zac was the assault he experienced when he was very young and conceptualised his depression, anxiety and other aspects of his distress as emanating from feelings he had not had opportunity to explore and express.

Louise was aware of some aspects of self-harm in Zac's narrative, including picking fights, 'reckless' behaviour and generalised suicidal thoughts. Louise was also aware of Zac alluding to 'other things' he did to cope, and talked through in supervision how she might explore this with him.

Sessions 2 and 3

Following discussion with her supervisor, Louise decided to ask Zac more about the 'other things' he did. She was aware of her temptation to avoid finding out more fearing what he might say, but also the danger of encouraging Zac to talk before he was ready. The dialogue that took place in Session 2 is outlined in Box 2.

Box 2: Louise's exploration with Zac about his coping strategies		
1	Louise:	When we met last week Zac you said there were other things you did to cope. I know it might be hard to talk about, but I wondered if you were able to tell me anything more about that?
2	Zac:	It's hard to say, y'know, cos I'm not sure about it really … about what you might think.
3	Louise:	We can all do things to cope with difficult feelings Zac. Sometimes we can hurt ourselves when the feelings are really bad, or really powerful. I'm not sure if how you feel ever gets that bad?
4	Zac:	Sometimes it does. Sometimes I feel so crap it's like it just builds up inside – like a real pressure, y'know. I just don't know where to go with it or what to do.
5	Louise:	So the crap just builds up inside … a real pressure?

6	Zac:	Yeah. I just have to do something with it or I think I will go mad.
7	Louise:	I suppose that's what I meant before about things we might do when we feel so bad. I wonder if you ever hurt yourself as a means of coping with your feelings?
8	Zac:	I do. Sometimes. I feel really strange telling you about it.
9	Louise:	I get it can be hard to talk about it. Do you want to tell me any more?
10	Zac:	Well, sometimes I cut myself, with a razor blade, y'know. Just a bit.
11	Louise	And how do you feel when you cut yourself?
12	Zac:	It's like a relief. Suddenly it eases off and I don't feel so bad, straight after.
13	Louise:	Cutting yourself relieves that build-up inside. How do you manage the cuts when you have done them?
14	Zac:	It's not too bad. Sometimes they're okay, and other times I look after them, keep them clean.
15	Louise:	So the bad ones you look after and make sure they're alright. It feels important to you to take care of them?
16	Zac:	I guess so. Sometimes it feels like the only time I take care of myself.

We can see a number of important therapeutic tasks going on here, with Louise using a number of skills, including reflection (lines 5, 13), summarising (line 15) and explorative statements (lines 3, 7 and 11). Often Louise links exploration with empathic responses, such as paraphrases or reflections, so that the questions remain anchored in the dialogue rather than coming from a point of wider curiosity.

In terms of Zac's self-harm Louise is also exploring issues of risk, determining the extent of Zac's harming, providing him with a space for self-**disclosure**, attending to possible feelings of shame and self-punishment, and opening other therapeutic doors for Zac should he wish to explore things more. What is important is that Louise's invitation to Zac to talk was tentative, but sufficiently grounded to communicate to him it was okay to do so. At line 2 or 4 Zac could have chosen not to disclose, and Louise would have respected his position.

How Louise and Zac respond to these opportunities in the relationship will be informed by the **relational** dynamic between them both, the modality of counselling, and Zac's goals. For example, from a CBT perspective support might focus on Zac's anxiety and how he views himself so negatively. He might work on his experience of himself in the 'now', working at changing aspects of how he thinks and behaves, and then how he feels. This may also include strategies to reduce his self-harm. Psychodynamically Zac may be encouraged by his therapist to explore the repressed feelings he holds unconsciously and understand his self-harm as an attack on himself, perhaps giving insight to his rage, for example. Humanistically Zac would be encouraged to tell his story, with the therapist reflecting to Zac aspects of his story and how he tells it. A natural question to ask Zac at the end of the dialogue above might be what he would like to do about his self-harm; this would be appropriate from any theoretical frame, as outlined in Box 3.

Box 3: Checking with the client focus for counselling

1	Louise:	That feels really important … what you say about taking care of yourself. Perhaps we can begin to think about other ways you might be able to take care of yourself too?
2	Zac:	Yeah, that would be a start.
3	Louise:	I also wonder Zac whether you want to spend any time looking at your self-harm in more detail, in terms of managing it differently, or understanding it more?
4	Zac:	We could. But I also think I do it cos of how crap I feel and I reckon that if I didn't feel quite so crap then I wouldn't do it anyway.
5	Louise:	So your cutting is a barometer of how bad you feel.
6	Zac:	Yeah. I suppose it is.
7	Louise:	OK. So let's continue to talk about how you feel and ways in which you might manage that differently for yourself. We can come back to the self-harm at any stage if that would be helpful.

The temptation for Louise, and any counsellor, would be to become self-harm focused. While there might be merit in focusing more on Zac's cutting in an attempt to find a way forward, the reality is that this is not a priority for Zac given how he understands what he does. What Louise does, however, is to introduce the concept of 'self-harm', ascertain Zac's level of self-understanding about what he does, re-focus the counselling and leave the door open to further exploration, if Zac wishes to.

Sessions 4 and 5

Louise's work with Zac continues to progress well. His anxiety reduces as he learns strategies for coping with high anxiety and panic, and his depression is less intense. Zac talked a little about the assault, for the first time, and found this particularly liberating. He reported his self-harm increased in frequency for a while and Louise and he were able to explore the reasons for this: that he was beginning to explore some of the internal feelings that contributed to him feeling 'crap' and, as such, was beginning to face some difficult things. In doing so his support strategies came to the fore which, in Zac's case, included cutting himself. Louise was able to help Zac integrate his behaviour (self-harm) with his narrative, which provided more opportunity for him to deal with it differently.

In session 4 Zac returned to his cutting specifically (as clients often will when given space and time to do so). He was interested in what his cutting really communicated. In integrating Zac's cutting into his wider story Louise made use of this as a strategy. Hill and Dallos (2011) undertook some interesting work on the narrative of self-harm. Their focus was about helping the client tell their story about self-harm, with the following recommendations:

- Counsellors should appreciate the importance of helping clients develop narratives around their self-harm.
- The counsellor's role is to be active in facilitating the client telling their story.
- The counsellor should encourage the client to include in their narrative speculations around meaning.
- The counsellor should avoid medicalising language or diagnostic terms as they can inhibit the story.
- The narrative can be used as a tool by the client to begin to see a different way of creating meaning: they can be facilitated to re-write their own story.

Louise and Zac agreed they would use Session 4 to help him talk about his self-harm. Louise reassured Zac there was no 'right' or 'wrong' way, but to talk as if the cuts, or the blade, had something to say. They agreed to audio-record part of the session and for Louise and Zac to select a small section to focus on. A small selection from the session is shown in Box 4.

Box 4: Zac's self-harm story

1	Zac:	It's like a can of fizzy drink… just ready to go bang but with nowhere to go. Just building up and building up and … and then there's the blood and in that moment I exist. It's like being able to breathe again and it's like my 'self' is just too big for my skin – releasing the pressure.
2	Louise:	In that moment you exist again.
3	Zac:	Yes. Yes I do. For all this time I feel there has been a big part of me hidden and invisible. All that time of hurting. And then I feel I exist again and I see the blood and it suddenly feels better. I feel better. In that moment I have nothing to feel ashamed about … doesn't haunt me anymore.
4	Louise:	Nothing to feel ashamed about … nothing to haunt you anymore.

In being invited to tell his story Zac is able to liberate himself from all expectations and fears of how he should be – the conditioning into emotional silence by being male, the shame of the assault, the burden of the secrets. It is a powerful story. Louise and Zac then restructure it into more of a stanza (poetry) format (without changing any of the words) to see how it reads:

It's like a can of fizzy drink,

just ready to go bang but

with nowhere to go.

Just

building up and

building up and

and then there's the blood and

in that moment

I exist.

It's like being able to breathe again and

It's like my 'self' is just too big for my skin

– releasing the pressure (In that moment you exist again)

Yes.

Yes, I do.

For all this time

I feel there has been a big part of me

hidden and invisible.

All that time of hurting.

And then I feel I exist again and

I see the blood

and it suddenly feels better.

I feel better.

In that moment

I have nothing to feel ashamed about.

Doesn't haunt me anymore.

(Nothing to feel ashamed about)

(Nothing to haunt you anymore)

Zac was profoundly moved when he read out his story as it appears above. He cried for the first time in many months but also felt enormously powerful because of some of the things he had said:

I exist; all that time of hurting; I feel better; I have nothing to feel ashamed about; and doesn't haunt me anymore.

This is a pivotal moment for Zac in being able to name things he had never mentioned before, and also in re-framing a sense of self that had otherwise eluded him. His self-harm had become a mechanism through which he could change and develop.

Session 6

Session 6 was the final session. Louise and Zac were able to review the work they had undertaken and Zac was encouraged to note what had changed. He felt significantly better about himself, his depression was much less intense, his anxiety reduced and his self-harm much less intense. Zac was no longer picking fights and was taking much greater care with himself. He had not cut himself since the last session, although the occasional urge to do so was sometimes there. Louise and Zac were able to acknowledge how hard it can be to leave behind a familiar way of doing things, and Zac felt that the purpose of his self-harm was no longer relevant. They both reflected on how Zac could continue to support himself in the future.

Summary

I have illustrated the value in working with the meaning of self-harm with clients. I am not suggesting that a narrative approach to such work is always the right option, or indeed the best option. In Chapter 6 we will consider different ways of working that might additionally be helpful, using a range of skills and ideas drawn from other modalities. However, the central point to be made here is that while particular skills and strategies might have value, being grounded in your work as a counsellor, utilising all that you do to develop, support, maintain and sustain therapeutic relationships is, above all, most important in working with self-harm.

Further reading

Reeves, A. & Howdin, J. (2010) *Considerations for Working with People Who Self-Harm,* Information Sheet G12. Lutterworth: BACP.

Turp, M. (2003) *Hidden Self-Harm. Narratives from Psychotherapy.* London: Jessica Kingsley.

Chapter 4
Identifying anxieties

There have been a number of occasions in my work with clients when I have been all too aware of the difference between discussing issues in the safety of the classroom or lecture theatre, and how they present in counselling. A good example is bereavement: we can read about stages of bereavement or continuing bonds theory and make sense of that in relation to our own experience. However, when sitting with a sobbing client at a point of despair when working through their grief, the chasm between an intellectual understanding of something and how it might present in reality is very stark. The same is true for working with self-harm: we may reflect on the definitions and types of behaviour as already outlined in the introductory chapter of this book from a particular perspective, but then be surprised by the visceral impact of a discourse about self-harm, or of a client describing their self-harm or showing the consequences of such.

Favazza (1989, p. 143) states that, 'Of all disturbing patient behaviours, self-mutilation is the most difficult for clinicians to understand and treat', and that counsellors can feel a range of responses to self-harm, including: sadness, anxiety, horror, helplessness, guilt, anger and disgust. These are powerful feelings and the temptation can be to try and disconnect from them, or 'leave them at the door' (the 'door' that counsellors so often wish to leave things at that might cause difficulty or challenge but, however successful they think they have been at doing so, never actually achieve).

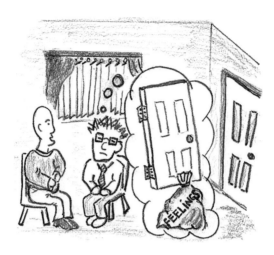

Figure 4.1 The counsellor leaves their feelings at the door

The reality is that all these feelings, and others, including empathy, warmth, compassion and hope, for example, are vital aspects of the therapeutic **process** and relationship. These need to be present, in some form or other, for the relationship to be based on a human exchange as opposed to an automated and enacted process of apparent 'caring'. That is, in being fully present with our clients we also need to be fully present to our responses to things they might do or say. This will be defined to some extent by our theoretical orientation and way of working. For example, a person-centred counsellor might, through a process of **congruence**, name their responses in a way helpful to the client, whereas a psychodynamic counsellor might keep such responses to themselves but instead offer interpretations of behaviour or actions. However, my assertion here is that, regardless of theoretical orientation, self-harm is still likely to impact on the humanity of the counsellor and thus the consequences of this will be present, in some form, in the therapeutic process.

To support this last point, research tells us a great deal about how self-harm can affect the counsellor. Sexton (1999) for example, outlines that counsellors can experience a loss of hope and cynicism in response to their client's self-harm, while Sanderson (2006) talks of the range of negative feelings counsellors can have, including a sense of personal and professional inadequacy and powerlessness. A relationship has been suggested between a counsellor's response to client self-harm and professional burn-out, compassion fatigue and vicarious traumatisation (Figley, 1995; Sexton, 1999; Pearlman and Saakvitne, 1995). Vicarious trauma can be defined as a, 'transformation in the helper's inner sense of identity and existence that results from utilising controlled empathy when listening to clients' trauma-content narratives. In other words, Vicarious Trauma is what happens to your neurological (or cognitive), physical, psychological, emotional and spiritual health when you listen to traumatic stories day after day or respond to traumatic situations while having to control your reaction.'

(www.vicarioustrauma.com/whatis.html, 2012)

Important here is the idea of 'utilising controlled empathy when listening to clients' trauma-content **narratives'** – that is, managing our visceral and felt response so that the client instead receives a controlled 'therapy' response.

I am not suggesting that the careful management of our responses is not a right, or indeed ethical, thing to do, given that an unmanaged response of disgust or horror at a client's narrative has the potential to cause enormous hurt and damage. Instead, it is important for us to explore how we might use our responses as a means of informing the counselling relationship and the client's understanding of their process rather than **dissociating** from responses, running the risk of simply offering anodyne or meaningless automated reactions that have the potential to leave the client feeling disconnected, unheard and on their own. Successful therapeutic work with self-harm might therefore take place in that middle ground, as outlined in Figure 4.2. To do this, however, we need to consider more carefully our anxieties about working with self-harm.

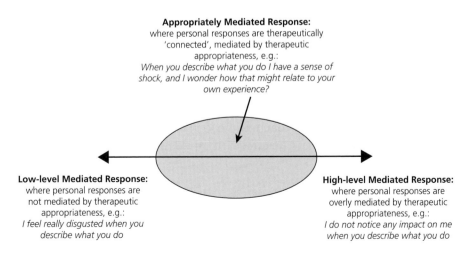

Appropriately Mediated Response:
where personal responses are therapeutically 'connected', mediated by therapeutic appropriateness, e.g.:
When you describe what you do I have a sense of shock, and I wonder how that might relate to your own experience?

Low-level Mediated Response:
where personal responses are not mediated by therapeutic appropriateness, e.g.:
I feel really disgusted when you describe what you do

High-level Mediated Response:
where personal responses are overly mediated by therapeutic appropriateness, e.g.:
I do not notice any impact on me when you describe what you do

Figure 4.2 A continuum of counsellor responses to self-harm

The nature of anxiety

There may be a number of anxieties aroused when working with self-harm in counselling. These might be split between: professional anxieties (framed within the context of our work as counsellors); process anxieties (concerns about what happens in the therapeutic relationship); and personal anxieties (framed within the context of a sense of self-integrity and self-experience). An outline of professional and personal anxieties appears below.

- **Professional**
  - Do I have the right training and experience to work with this client?
  - Should I be talking to anyone else about my client's self-harm if I am concerned?
  - Should I be referring my client to another counsellor/service because of their self-harm?
  - What if my organisational setting has a policy about working with self-harm?
- **Process**
  - What if self-harm gets worse while my client is in counselling?
  - How can I best talk about self-harm with my client?
  - Self-harm and suicide seem to be related. How will I know my client will not kill themselves?
  - If we talk about self-harm will that make matters worse?
- **Personal**
  - Deep down I really do not understand it, or 'approve' of it. What can I do?
  - What if I relate to or identify with a client's experience?
  - I do not have a strong stomach: talking in detail about self-harm frightens me.
  - Is what I can offer going to be enough?

It will be helpful to elaborate on each of these in turn in the context of a case scenario that illustrates how our anxieties might be raised during the counselling process.

Professional

Do I have the right training and experience to work with this client?

> # Voices
> ....
>
> ## Eleanor
> Eleanor is 17 years old and attends a young person's counselling agency. She sees a counsellor for an assessment session and then is allocated to Zara, a trainee counsellor who works in the agency on placement. While Eleanor was asked about self-harm during assessment, she did not disclose any. During her work with Zara she begins to talk about how she has cut herself on her arms for 'a couple of years'. Zara feels frightened and unsure about how to work with Eleanor because of this new **disclosure**.

Working ethically means, amongst other things, working within our own limits of knowledge and skills. Any one of us can feel anxiety when faced with a client whose difficulties and distress fall outside of our own immediate knowledge or experience. For many counsellors the presence of a discussion of self-harm in counselling can be experienced as difficult. This is true of both qualified and trainee counsellors alike and we can quickly be transported to a place where we either doubt our own competence to work with self-harm, or believe ourselves to be incompetent to do so. This might be because we simply do not have the knowledge or understanding to conceptualise why someone might harm themselves and feel panicky in response to such a disclosure, or it might be that we fear that will be the case.

Zara's experience in the scenario above will mirror many people's experience in training. However careful initial assessments are, clients may choose not to disclose information about self-harm at that point, only doing so when they feel sufficiently safe with a counsellor. It is therefore not uncommon for trainee counsellors to find themselves working with a client who later discloses self-harm. Zara immediately feels frightened (by the possibility she might 'get it wrong' perhaps), and doubts her competence to offer Eleanor the type of support she needs. The temptation is to withdraw from the counselling relationship as quickly as possible. However, it is likely that Eleanor has disclosed self-harm to Zara for the very fact that she feels comfortable and safe with her. There is sufficient trust in Zara, as well as a sufficiently grounded therapeutic relationship, to facilitate Eleanor's increased honesty about her distress.

In this particular scenario Zara discussed her concerns in supervision and was able to better understand the particular aspects of Eleanor's disclosure that frightened her the most and, in doing so, felt better able to re-connect with Eleanor and the therapeutic process. This provided Eleanor with the space she needed to explore her difficulties fully. Zara was surprised, when reflecting on the relationship after she had finished working with Eleanor, that self-harm was not the real focus of the work and improved as Eleanor felt stronger. Zara had begun a process of building competency and experience in working with self-harm. However, if following supervision Zara had not felt able to work with Eleanor it would have been right for her to arrange for a re-referral, managing this appropriately for Eleanor.

Should I be talking to anyone else about my client's self-harm if I am concerned?

Voices

Frank

Frank works as a newly qualified counsellor in an education setting. He sees Paula, a 16-year-old student who has been talking about her self-harm for several sessions. She has burnt herself with cigarettes for a few months, but has also recently started to engage in sexually risky behaviour, going home with strangers for sex.

When we contract with clients at the beginning of counselling we typically place limits on confidentiality boundaried by risk to self or others. For the most part we are able to work within those boundaries and do not have to worry about whether or not to discuss our concerns about a client with someone else. The disclosure of self-harm may be something we think about in relation to the boundaries we have agreed and, again for the most part, we are able to work within our boundaries of confidentiality in a safe and ethical manner.

Frank's work with Paula has been going well, and they both feel she has been making progress. The agency in which Frank works has a policy on self-harm that states that where self-harm is seen to escalate or seriously change in nature the counsellor should consult the manager. Frank and Paula have discussed her self-burning and have been exploring the meaning of this for Paula. As a result Paula has been burning herself less and is feeling a little stronger. However, Frank also recognises Paula's sexual risk-taking as a form of self-harming too, and raises this thought with Paula. She understands Frank's concern and acknowledges that she feels like she is 'spiralling out of control'.

In Frank's scenario he is working well with Paula but is also identifying increased risk. His question, to be further explored in supervision and with his manager, is whether counselling is sufficient support for Paula in itself or whether, with Paula's consent, he might access other support on her behalf. This question relates not only to the one on competency we discussed earlier, but also to whether counselling can meet Paula's needs on its own.

We might often think about a range of behaviours and actions that might fall beyond our own capacity to work with someone, and might additionally be uncertain as to the boundary between self-harm as a survival mechanism, and when self-harm changes and becomes increasingly threatening to the client's well-being. Frank has to carefully balance the successes Paula has been making in reducing the frequency and severity of her self-burning, weighing this against the fact that she is beginning to self-harm in different ways, with different dangers. Whether we share concerns about risk to self and how we go about it are difficult ethical dilemmas.

Should I be referring my client to another counsellor/service because of their self-harm?

Voices

Duncan

Duncan has been working with Antony for several months, offering counselling to help Antony with concerns he has about low self-esteem and poor body image. Antony came to counselling because he had started to use performance enhancing drugs as part of what was already excessive gym use. Antony had recognised for himself that he was starting to get out of his 'depth' and saw counselling as a positive way of dealing with his worries. However, while Antony understands himself more, he has started using other drugs and fears that he is losing control of his life.

While it may be possible to identify a number of clear areas of focus early on in counselling, either through assessment or early exploration, it is very common for these areas of focus – or client goals – to change during the course of therapy. The need to regularly review counselling with clients is highlighted here, with the benefit of ensuring that counselling continues to meet the changing needs clients may experience. The same is true with self-harm, where a client may present with an underlying problem (low self-esteem and poor body image for Antony), and specific additional issues relating to it (the use of performance enhancing drugs as a means to deal with a 'poor body', as opposed to dealing with the real problem: poor body-image).

While the work was progressing well, with Antony feeling a little more confident about himself, Duncan is now anxious that Antony's self-harm is beginning to change so that the support he requires is also changing. Duncan is particularly concerned about Antony's increasing drug use and his fears of losing control over his life, but also notes the value Antony places on the therapeutic relationship and the trust he seems to have in Duncan. The difficulty here is whether to refer Antony on to another, more specialised, service, to continue to work with the issue in counselling, or both. How, when or if Duncan explores this with Antony is difficult, as Duncan does not want to communicate that he no longer wishes to be involved in the relationship.

What if my organisational setting has a policy about working with self-harm?

Voices

Francine

Francine is a counsellor working for a bereavement agency. She works with Edward who is 54 years old. His partner died in a road traffic accident 12 months previously and Edward has struggled to manage his grief. At times he feels quite overwhelmed and discloses to Francine that while he used to hit and punch himself when frustrated, since the death of his partner he has been cutting himself with a kitchen knife. The organisation in which Francine works has a policy which states that the client's GP should be contacted about all clients who are at risk to themselves.

Working in any organisational setting, as we will explore in the next chapter, demands that we pay careful attention to any policies, procedures and guidance about how to work with particular issues. It is not uncommon for organisations to have a risk policy, which usually relates to harm to self or others (amongst other aspects). While for the most part such policies are in place to guide counsellors in their work and to ensure the most vulnerable clients are responded to appropriately, sometimes policies are a means of organisations responding to their own anxieties about risk. It is important to note here that anxieties can be held not only by individual practitioners, but also by the organisations in which they work, who fear the consequence of a serious incident, such as a client death.

Francine has a very difficult dilemma, the nature of which we will discuss more in the chapter on ethical issues (Chapter 8). In this instance, however, Francine has to manage her work with Edward, who has placed trust in her to the point where he feels able to disclose very difficult things, against the organisation's policy which seems to direct Francine to speak to Edward's GP. This scenario raises an important dilemma of uncertainty about risk that counsellors are often concerned about. As with many policies on risk, a course of action is outlined, but the particular triggers that would lead to a course of action are not defined. For Francine, she has to make a decision, ideally in collaboration with Edward, about whether his recent self-harming behaviour represents a 'risk to self' or whether instead it is a way in which Edward is coping in the short-term, which counselling may be able to help address.

Process

What if self-harm gets worse while my client is in counselling?

Voices

Annette

Annette, who is 42 years old, has been seeing her counsellor for several months. She was referred by her GP following a long period of depression. She has been finding counselling with Georgina, her counsellor, extremely helpful and has taken the opportunity to talk about a number of problems. These have included her experiences of abuse while growing up, periods of time in local authority care and what she describes as 'general chaos'. She has self-harmed by cutting herself for some years.

Self-harm can have a profound effect on both the client and counsellor during the process of therapy. It is very easy as a counsellor to become self-harm focussed, so that the action of self-harm becomes the primary focal point for counselling with all attempts made to help the client stop. Unconsciously self-harm can become a barometer by which the 'success' of counselling is judged, perhaps by counsellor and client alike: if the client stops self-harming then counselling is 'successful', whereas if self-harm increases or continues, counselling is 'unsuccessful'. This is a very unhelpful way of viewing self-harm and is more about the counsellor's need than the client's.

In Annette's scenario, it would be easy for Georgina to focus on Annette's self-harm, her cutting, without paying attention to the wider **narrative**. However, it is also important that Georgina does not make quick assumptions about the nature of self-harm (for example, that Annette self-harms because of abuse). We can be tempted to either jump to conclusions about causality, or instead focus only on specific behaviour.

How can I best talk about self-harm with my client?

Voices

William

William is a 22-year-old client who has started counselling because of anger. He reports to his counsellor, Tanya, that he regularly gets into fights (often provoking them himself) and is regularly injured because of them. He drinks heavily and has a poor relationship with his family. He has a small group of friends, who stand by him, but many others find him too aggressive; he feels quite lonely.

It is unusual for a client to come to counselling specifically because of self-harm, with the sole focus of talking about self-harm. While this does occasionally happen, it is more typical for clients to talk about a range of problems and difficulties where self-harm is one of them. As we have discussed previously, the temptation to be drawn to discussing self-harm can be strong. Instead, counselling needs to follow the focus and goals of the counselling, which might be about exploring a range of other issues and, often, might not include discussing the self-harm at all.

However, it can be equally unhelpful for the counsellor to avoid any discussion about the client's self-harm, as this can communicate disinterest, or that self-harm is something best not talked about. In supervision,

Tanya has begun to see William's fighting as a form of self-harm, in which he sustains injuries albeit not inflicted directly by himself. His repeating pattern of getting into harmful fights is not dissimilar to him injuring himself directly. Tanya's anxiety centres on how, or whether, to make this link in counselling. She fears that by suggesting William's behaviour is a form of self-harm she might cause more upset, or make matters worse.

Self-harm and suicide seem to be related. How will I know my client will not kill themselves?

Voices

Liam

Liam has been in contact with mental health support services for several years. He experienced early onset **psychosis** and was referred to an **Early Intervention Team** and responded well to their support. He was prescribed medication by his psychiatrist and was also referred to counselling, where he now sees Andrew. Liam's mental health has deteriorated over recent months, but his psychiatrist still wants to avoid a hospital admission for Liam. Liam has started to take initially small overdoses of his medication, necessitating treatment in A&E.

As we have discussed already, the term 'risk to self' when setting boundaries around confidentiality is insufficiently defined and, as a consequence, has the potential to bring any range of behaviours into the range of a counsellor's anxiety. For many clients, self-harm will be a mechanism through which they self-support and thus lessen the chance of further increased harm or suicide. However, there may also be instances when a client's actions, while intended as a mechanism of self-harm, have the potential to lead to a different outcome, including the client's death.

Andrew and Liam have talked about Liam's overdosing as a form of self-harm. Liam does not intend to die by taking an overdose of his medication and seeks further assistance quickly, but the process of taking the overdose and the subsequent treatment in A&E forms part of his self-harming process. Andrew is concerned about the effects of the repeated overdoses on Liam and that Liam seems to be taking more tablets on each occasion. Liam is reluctant for Andrew to talk about his concerns to the psychiatrist as Liam wishes to avoid a hospital admission. It is a difficult dilemma for Andrew in knowing how safe Liam will continue to be and at what point he should raise his concerns with others, without Liam's consent if necessary.

If we talk about self-harm will that make matters worse?

Voices

Bonnie

Bonnie is a counsellor working in a voluntary sector agency which offers generic counselling to any adult free of charge. She has been seeing Doreen for several weeks. Doreen is in a violent relationship and feels unable to leave. She has been drinking heavily to cope and has alluded to 'other things' she does, without going into detail.

One of the biggest fears when working with risk, whether suicide or self-harm, is that by talking about it the risk will be increased. The fear is that the naming of self-harm and subsequent exploration of it has the potential to make it more 'concrete' and real to the client, thus reinforcing their actions and contributing to the maintenance of harmful behaviour.

Bonnie has been anxious about Doreen's situation since they first met, but has felt preoccupied by Doreen's comments about the 'other things' she does to cope. She has discussed this in supervision and has been encouraged by her supervisor to explore this phrase with Doreen in more detail, offering her an opportunity to name more specifically what she means and what implications this may have for her safety and well-being. Bonnie, however, remains very anxious about doing so for fear of making matters worse.

Personal

Deep down I really do not understand it, or 'approve' of it. What can I do?

Voices

Joyce

Joyce is a 34-year-old newly qualified counsellor. During her placement she did not knowingly work with any client who self-harmed, but has recently been referred a new client, Dawn, who has written on her registration form that she 'cuts' herself when she feels 'really bad'. Joyce has already noticed a very strong reaction in herself, feeling angry towards Dawn. She simply wants to tell Dawn to 'stop it', but knows she cannot do that.

As counsellors we are challenged often to reflect on our own position about particular things, particularly when they relate to why a client has come to counselling. Our own views about things, based on our own experience or faith-based views for example, all have the potential to be present in counselling if we are not actively aware of them and do not manage them accordingly. As we have discussed, it is not uncommon for self-harm to provoke such responses in counsellors.

While Joyce has not met Dawn yet, she has already noticed a number of strong reactions in herself and is caught in a dilemma where she wants to act on her feelings, but knows it would be unhelpful or inappropriate to do so. Joyce's challenge here is to explore the source of her strong responses and, if they cannot be mitigated by increased self-awareness, to find a way of supporting herself so that she can continue to work effectively with Dawn; otherwise Dawn might be better seeing another counsellor.

What if I relate to or identify with a client's experience?

Voices

Deshi

Deshi became a counsellor following her own positive experience of therapy. She had struggled with depression and self-harm herself for several years and had attended counselling on the advice of a friend. While she knows counselling is not for everyone, she still feels that most people could benefit from it, based on her own experience. She has been meeting with Victoria who, while she experiences depression and also self-harms, is very hesitant about counselling.

It can always pose difficulties in counselling when working with a client whose experiences relate closely to our own. The danger of **identification**, rather than empathy, can cloud both our judgement and focus. It is also worth noting that the concept of **transference** (where the client unconsciously transfers **relational** experiences from previous relationships into the therapeutic relationship) is important. While transference is typically associated with psychoanalytic or psychodynamic models specifically, the concept is arguably relevant for all our work, regardless of orientation. This is also true for **countertransference** (the counsellor's unconscious responses to the client that are shaped by experiences and relationships outside the therapeutic process). Taken together, transference and countertransference (or however we might chose to name these dynamics) will also inform the process with clients who self-harm. I will discuss this in more depth in the chapter on therapeutic techniques (Chapter 5). Without realising, we can be drawn into helping ourselves, rather than remaining client-focussed.

Deshi is already aware of her powerful allegiance to counselling because of how it had helped her at times of difficulty. Victoria poses a particular challenge for her in that on hearing her story Deshi realises that she can relate to much of what Victoria is saying, including about self-harm. The specific challenge is two-fold: first, in not pushing Victoria, who is uncertain about counselling, further and faster than Victoria might ordinarily be willing to go; second, to not conflate Victoria's and her own experience and thus act on her own feelings rather than remaining focused on Victoria's.

I do not have a strong stomach: talking in detail about self-harm frightens me

Voices

Sally-Ann

Sally-Ann, a counsellor working in a university setting, works with Adrian, a 19-year-old student who pulls his own hair, picks his skin and picks at scabs. While he is coping academically, Adrian struggles socially and feels very isolated. Sally-Ann experiences Adrian as a warm, compassionate and vulnerable young man, but finds it difficult to hear his accounts of self-harm.

We can internalise a number of perceived messages about how counsellors *should* be: strong; invincible; always prepared; knowing; compassionate and unshockable. On one hand we might be pleased to possess all these qualities, on the other being like this might take away one important component of being a good counsellor – being fallible. While we need to be strong-*enough* to contain and work with our client's distress, I would argue that **relational** depth is partly achieved through our **capacity** to be fallible and imperfect with our clients.

Sally-Ann has a dilemma: on one hand she feels very positively about Adrian while, on the other (if she were entirely honest with herself), she feels a little disgusted when he talks about his self-harm. She knows that she does not feel disgusted *with* Adrian, but rather about some of the things he says he does. She certainly does not wish to cause him distress or hurt, but also finds her reaction in sessions very hard to contain.

Is what I can offer going to be enough?

Voices

Clare

Clare is a person-centred counsellor who works with young care-leavers. She thoroughly enjoys her work and feels that counselling offers clients an invaluable space to learn about themselves. She also passionately believes that person-centred counselling is of particular value with this client group as they have had little opportunity to set the direction of their own life. Clare notices, however, that when working with clients who self-harm she doubts the value of her work and often thinks that someone else would be able to help the client more effectively than her.

It is not uncommon for us to assume, particularly when working with a client who has complex or challenging experiences, that someone else (*anyone else!*) would be a more effective helper than ourselves. The temptation to pass on the 'hot potato' (that is, the challenging **narrative** rather than the client themselves) can be high. In the face of adversity we can lose confidence in our own **capacity** to care or to be able to offer the client the safe, respectful and confidential space they need.

Clare is committed both to her work as a counsellor and also to the value of her model of counselling in the context in which she works. While she does not doubt the efficacy or benefits of other models, she feels that specifically for her client group – care-leavers – the non-directive nature of her work helps them begin to take control over their lives. However, she feels that she ought to be able to 'do more' when working with self-harm and someone else would probably have better insight into self-harm and know more strategies to help them stop.

Reflective task

Consider the scenarios outlined throughout this chapter. Select three or four that might cause you the most concern. Write a list of the specific things that worry you most about each scenario – be as detailed as you can. How do you feel about the scenarios and the anxieties you have listed and, having completed the list, what active steps could you take to support yourself? That is, what are your solutions?

Summary

In this chapter I have outlined a number of common, and shared, anxieties when working with clients who self-harm. Before moving on later in the book to consider possible resolutions to these anxieties, it is important not to rush on from them either. Counsellors can often experience enormous guilt at not being perfect, instead feeling things they would rather not: like a guilty secret. However, underlying all these anxieties is the fact that they are all also very human, reasonable, understandable and appropriate. It is not having anxiety that is the challenge, but rather knowing ourselves enough to recognise and give permission to our anxieties. It is this that will best place us to work with them effectively in our work.

Further reading

Fleet, D. & Mintz, R. (2012) 'Counsellors' perceptions of client progression when working with clients who intentionally self-harm and the impact such work has on the therapist'. *Counselling and Psychotherapy Research*. **www.tandfonline.com/doi/abs/10.1080/14733145.2012.69 8421** pp. 1–9.

Reeves, A. (2012) 'Working with suicide and self-harm in counselling', in C Feltham and I Horton (eds) *The SAGE Handbook of Counselling and Psychotherapy* London: Sage, pp 539–33.

Chapter 5
Strategies for the management of anxieties

We have previously identified a number of anxieties that counsellors may experience when working with clients who self-harm. We categorised them into three groups: professional anxieties; **process** anxieties; and personal anxieties. This is because different aspects of our work with clients will impact on us in different ways. We may, for example, have concerns about a client's well-being or safety, or perhaps about how the therapeutic relationship is progressing or whether it is progressing as it should, or instead about our own feelings and responses when faced with the reality of self-harm.

Having identified these anxieties, the purpose of this chapter is to consider in more detail how we might respond to them. This might involve professional actions, ways in which we might respond therapeutically or around self-care. I will revisit these three categories here using the same case scenarios we identified earlier to consider how the counsellors might work actively on finding strategies to support themselves and their work.

Professional

Do I have the right training and experience to work with this client?

Voices

Eleanor

Eleanor is 17 years old and attends a young person's counselling agency. She sees a counsellor for an assessment session and is then allocated to Zara, a trainee counsellor, who works in the agency on placement. When Eleanor was asked about self-harm during assessment, she did not disclose any. During her work with Zara she begins to talk about how she has cut herself on her arms for 'a couple of years'. Zara feels frightened and unsure about how to work with Eleanor because of this new **disclosure**.

When a client discloses self-harm during counselling, perhaps because it was not known about previously because it had not been talked about at referral or during assessment, it can throw both counsellor and client into a state of confusion. It can be experienced as such a 'big' disclosure (that is, something of apparent overriding importance), that the other work becomes overshadowed by it. This may also parallel how the client feels; that their self-harm has become the mechanism through which all their distress is experienced so that the detail of their struggle is overshadowed by their actions at times of acute difficulty.

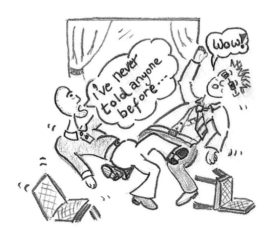

Figure 5.1 A big disclosure can throw both the client and counsellor into a state of confusion

The temptation for Zara therefore, is to become self-harm-focused, centring in on the new disclosure believing it inevitably to be the important area for the client. Or, at the other end of the scale, Zara might avoid the new disclosure, unsure about whether or how to respond. The reality is that the **disclosure** of self-harm is important because the client has introduced it into the therapeutic frame. This may not necessarily be more or less important than anything else the client has explored. The task here for Zara is to acknowledge Eleanor's disclosure, perhaps discussing it in more detail as to when it began, when it happens now, how she feels about it, how she takes care of the injuries and herself, and what prompted the disclosure now. This would provide both Eleanor and Zara with an opportunity to find out more about the meaning and impact of Eleanor's self-harm and it would communicate to Eleanor that it is okay for her to talk about this. It would also provide Zara with an opportunity to understand the severity or otherwise of Eleanor's cutting, keeping an eye on risk.

Equally important, however, talking with Eleanor about her self-harm would provide an opportunity to explore whether her self-harm is to be the focus of the counselling. We might assume that more often than not, the client instead wants help with the causes of their distress, rather than how that distress presents. It might be that Eleanor wants her self-harming to be the focus of the work, but it might also be that Eleanor simply wants Zara to know about it, without it becoming the focus. Going back to the point above about a parallel process, there may be an important therapeutic benefit in Zara giving Eleanor implicit 'permission' to talk about how she feels, becoming less self-harm-focused herself.

Should I be talking to anyone else about my client's self-harm if I am concerned?

Voices

Frank

Frank works as a newly qualified counsellor in an education setting. He sees Paula, a 16-year-old student who has been talking about her self-harm for several sessions. She has burnt herself with cigarettes for a few months, but has also recently started to engage in sexually risky behaviour, going home with unknown people for sex.

Working within our own competence is an ethical requirement under most professional codes or frameworks for good practice. It is important not to work beyond our skills, knowledge and training. Any counsellor who discusses in supervision, or with their line manager, that they feel out of their depth in work with a client should either be supported to help develop understanding or competence, or encouraged to discuss with the client other possible options of support.

It is not uncommon, however, for counsellors to feel out of their depth simply following a disclosure of self-harm. It may be that the therapeutic relationship has otherwise been experienced by counsellor and client alike as facilitative, supportive and helpful. But, following the disclosure of self-harm, or when self-harm is part of the client's **narrative**, the counsellor may assume the work is beyond what they can manage.

In this scenario Frank feels out of his depth as a relatively newly qualified counsellor and thinks he should be talking to someone else, beyond line management support and supervision, about helping Paula. His position is that he, as her counsellor, is insufficient to meet her needs. However, Frank is also aware that, as Paula is 16, there are **safeguarding** issues for him to consider also. Safeguarding refers to policies and procedures, typically in place in settings where the work is with young people or children, such as schools counselling, that attend to the safety and well-being of the young person or child. Safeguarding includes child protection (where specific harm is suspected), but also has wider terms that include more general safety. Frank's anxiety is therefore twofold: whether he is competent to work with Paula; and whether he has further safeguarding responsibilities that must also be attended to.

Almost all counsellors in the UK, if they are members of a professional organisation, have an ethical responsibility to be appropriately supervised for their work with clients. This is not a **statutory** responsibility, but rather one that members of professional organisations 'sign up' to on becoming a member. With supervision in place therefore, Frank's first step is to take his concerns to his supervisor. In supervision he will be supported in his work, will have opportunity to reflect on skills and knowledge that might inform his practice and, specifically in this scenario, will be given space to talk through Paula's well-being and whether he needs to act as a safeguarding requirement. The message here is that whilst we undertake our work with clients in a one-to-one format (typically), we should not consider ourselves to be alone and unsupported in reflecting on challenging and difficult situations.

There is no 'blueprint' for counsellors to work to that will help Frank with such difficult decisions. Instead, Frank needs to feel able to talk to his supervisor and line manager about his concerns and, following such discussions, talk more with Paula about possibilities of support and action so that any decision is, wherever possible, a collaborative one between counsellor and client. This best supports ongoing work with clients and facilitates them taking responsibility for their own well-being.

Should I be referring my client to another counsellor/service because of their self-harm?

Voices

Duncan

Duncan has been working with Antony for several months, offering counselling to help Antony with concerns he has about low self-esteem and poor body image. Antony came to counselling because he had started to use performance-enhancing drugs as part of what was already excessive gym use. Antony had recognised for himself that he was starting to get out of his 'depth' and saw counselling as a positive way of dealing with his worries. However, while Antony is understanding himself more, he has started using other drugs and fears that he is losing control of his life.

As we have already outlined in Frank's scenario, working within our competence is an ethical requirement for good practice in counselling. Duncan has been working with Antony for several months and, for the most part, the work has been experienced by Antony as helpful. He has achieved much more insight into the cause and nature of his problems but, at the same time, has continued to struggle with them. The work with Antony has been less about his use of performance-enhancing drugs (the behavioural response to his concerns), but instead about what Antony thinks about himself and his body and the development of these feelings (the cause of his distress).

This has been an insightful, but also difficult, process for Antony, as he has begun to address deep-seated feelings about himself. While his previous attempts to address his body image concerns have been responded to by Antony trying to change his body to make it 'better' and 'more accept-able' to others, Antony is now exploring the real nature of his hurt. As a consequence, Antony has started to try to 'anaesthetise' his feelings through the use of other drugs. They make him happy temporarily, but Antony also understands the more serious dangers that they bring.

Duncan is, understandably and rightly, reflecting on his level of competence to work with Antony's increasing drug use. Like the earlier scenario with Eleanor, however, the task is for Duncan to explore fully with Antony the nature of the drug use, its extent and his perceived control over it, and whether it has now become the focus for Antony. It may be that Antony has mentioned his drug use because he wants Duncan to know about it, but does not necessarily want it to become the focus of counselling (at this stage). If that were the case, it would provide Duncan with an opportunity to help Antony understand the function that drugs have for him, (stopping him from feeling), which might be more facilitative longer term and give Antony choices about what he might do differently.

However, it might be that Antony feels that he needs immediate and specific help with his escalating drug use, even though he understands what it means for him. In that instance it might be that Duncan has the skills and knowledge to support Antony with that or, following discussion in supervision, a better discussion with Antony would be about possible referral routes to agencies with the appropriate skills and resources to help Antony address the drug problem. This outcome would only become clearer through an open and honest dialogue between Duncan and Antony, which would be respectful of Duncan's confidence and competency as a counsellor, as well as identifying the most appropriate support needs for Antony and responding accordingly.

What if my organisational setting has a policy about working with self-harm?

Voices

Francine

Francine is a counsellor working for a bereavement agency. She works with Edward who is 54 years old. His partner died in a road traffic accident 12 months previously and Edward has struggled to manage his grief. At times he feels quite overwhelmed and **discloses** to Francine that while he used to hit and punch himself when frustrated, since the death of his partner he has been cutting himself with a kitchen knife. The organisation in which Francine works has a policy which states that the client's GP should be contacted about all clients who are at risk to themselves.

In working with any situation where risk is an inherent aspect, such as suicide potential, risk to others, or self-harm, it is the shades of grey that often cause the greatest anxiety. For example, where there is no risk, there is no anxiety about risk. Where the risk is so high (for example, where suicide potential is immediate), the contract we have with our clients and organisational policy usually requires us to act to try to safeguard the immediate well-being of the client. However, when we are uncertain about the nature and extent of the risk, we are left unsure about what, if anything, we should be doing in response.

Francine is aware of her organisation's policy about risk, in that where risk is evident, she has a duty under the policy to talk to the client's GP (presumably without the client's consent, if necessary – Francine would have to clarify this to ensure she was clear exactly what she would be expected to do so that she could ensure her client was also fully aware of this policy at the commencement of counselling). Edward has talked about other self-harm (hitting and punching himself) and Francine has made a judgement that while this is important information for her and Edward to explore, his actions do not place him in immediate risk of death and therefore Francine feels comfortable in keeping this information confidential. Edward's new **disclosure** about 'cutting himself with a kitchen knife' has, however, raised greater concerns for Francine and caused her to reconsider what she should do. Francine has a duty to explore in more detail with Edward what this means in reality for him.

As counsellors we must be aware of the danger of overreacting, or reacting too quickly, to information that immediately sounds dramatic or worrying but might, in actual fact, be less concerning once we know more. For example, the image that might be provoked for Francine of Edward causing himself severe or life-threatening damage with a long, sharp and dangerous kitchen knife would understandably cause her to be anxious. If, following discussion with Edward, it transpires that her image proved to reflect the actual situation then it may be appropriate to talk with Edward about the need for further assessment and support and the requirement to follow the terms of the organisational policy. However, it might also be that the 'kitchen knife' is a knife used for eating and Edward's actions constitute scratching himself. While this information would still be extremely important for Francine and Edward to talk more about, it would not constitute the same level of risk as would be apparent in the first scenario.

Following Edward's disclosure Francine could gently ask Edward, 'Can you tell me a bit more about what you do? What is the knife like and how and where do you harm yourself?'. Depending on his responses she can then ask more questions, or facilitate Edward in talking more about this. The important message here is that clear and factual information is key in determining how we might respond to clients in line with organisational expectations. The danger here is of responding to our worst fears. Talking to clients, however, openly and honestly, about what they have said will always facilitate a better and more informed outcome.

Process

What if self-harm gets worse while my client is in counselling?

Voices

Annette

Annette, who is 42 years old, has been seeing her counsellor for several months. She was referred by her GP following a long period of depression. She has been finding counselling with Georgina, her counsellor, extremely helpful and has taken the opportunity to talk about a number of problems. These have included her experiences of abuse while growing up, periods of time in local authority care and what she describes as 'general chaos'. She has self-harmed by cutting herself for some years.

When a client presents in counselling, our hope is that we will be able to help them feel better, whatever their source of distress. It is often not possible to judge whether our client is feeling 'better' beyond how they describe their experience of themselves. Sometimes clients make real progress but their experience of themselves is the opposite – the therapeutic task may be to challenge their self-perception with contradictory evidence to try and help them re-evaluate themselves. The other way in which we might be able to judge 'progress' is if we use outcome measures in a session (such as a 'tick-box' form the client completes session by session, or at frequent intervals, that measures change). Again however, such measures do not always reflect the nature of change that is occurring.

There may be particular aspects of the client's presentation that give us some clue to progress, such as when certain reported feelings or behaviours seem less prominent, although we are generally cautious about reading too much into this. When working with self-harm, however, we can often lock on to the action of self-harm and, consciously or unconsciously, begin to use it as a barometer of change. When self-harm seems to be improving we can interpret it as 'successful' counselling, and when it is getting worse or remaining unchanged we can then interpret that as 'unsuccessful' counselling. The danger, like many of the scenarios outlined already in this chapter, is to become too self-harm focused, missing other more important aspects of the client's experience.

As counsellors we must be very aware of the dangers of being drawn into seeing our client's self-harm as a barometer of the success of what we are offering, as this can happen very easily and quickly, even for the most experienced practitioners. The reality is that, for some clients, self-harm may get worse during the early stages of counselling. If we imagine self-harm as a means through which clients cope with or express difficult feelings, an increased awareness of those feelings can lead them to increased use of coping strategies, even if those coping strategies are harmful. As clients begin to talk about difficult or painful feelings in counselling they become more in touch with those feelings and, in such circumstances, will draw more on the ways in which they have coped until now.

The task, therefore, is to be open to a discussion at any stage with our clients about their self-harm and, particularly when self-harm remains an ongoing dynamic, to help clients to understand the function self-harm serves in how they cope. As counselling continues and, hopefully, more self-caring strategies are identified and practised, the self-harm is likely to reduce and then stop. The point here is that self-harm is replaced by self-care, which can be modelled by the counsellor. Annette's counselling with Georgina has been helpful and there is sufficient trust in the relationship for them to talk about Annette's self-harm. Annette can be supported by Georgina in understanding the function her self-harm has in managing feelings related to her abuse and upbringing and how they converge in her depression, so that should her self-harm remain or, for a short-time, get worse, this can be understood and thus less frightening. Clearly it would be important for Georgina to work with Annette to keep the extent of self-harm in focus so that any emerging issues of risk can be responded to.

How can I best talk about self-harm with my client?

Voices

William

William is a 22-year-old man who has started counselling because of anger. He reports to his counsellor, Tanya, that he regularly gets into fights (often provoking them himself) and is regularly injured because of them. He drinks heavily and has a poor relationship with his family. He has a small group of friends who stand by him, but many others find him too aggressive; he feels quite lonely.

William is very unhappy and has described a number of situations that are causing him particular difficulty, including self-harm (provoking fights that often result in injury). He also recognises feelings that underpin these actions, including anger and loneliness. In supervision, Tanya has been supported by her supervisor to understand William's fighting as a form of self-harm; he deliberately gets into fights that might serve an unconscious need for him to suffer pain and hurt which, in turn, become an expression of his anger and possible low self-esteem. Tanya's anxiety, however, is that William has not talked of the fights as self-harm and she is uncertain how she might introduce this into the counselling dialogue in a way that is helpful, or that does not cause harm. The danger is that Tanya avoids her anxiety by avoiding the things that are causing anxiety: naming William's actions as self-harming and being honest and possibly challenging with him.

The reality is, however, that William has come to counselling to help address his feelings and repeated harmful actions so that he can feel less angry, happier and thus function more successfully in his world; ultimately so that he feels less lonely and more connected with others in respectful and non-harmful ways. Counselling, possibly unlike any other relation-ship in his life, is a chance for William to explore his feelings openly and receive honest and constructive responses from another person. It might be that no-one else in William's life is prepared to say things to him that might really help.

Tanya's task therefore, and the one most likely to bring about positive change for William (and help Tanya address her own anxieties) is to talk to William openly about her thoughts. Clearly there are important cave-ats here in that Tanya needs to do so empathically, without judgement and in a way that William can 'hear' and make use of. Being gentle but not overly tentative might really enable William to be 'heard' himself. Tanya might say something like, 'I wondered about whether getting into fights was a way in which you harm yourself William? Instead of doing it directly to yourself the harm happens by others, but following fights you have provoked'. This may be challenging for William in that Tanya is bringing something about his behaviour from the edge of his awareness into his awareness. He can think about what Tanya has suggested and either reject it (as is his right), or accept it and use that new knowledge to understand what he does and why he does it a little more. Such honesty that is respectfully offered can really facilitate a therapeutic **process** and demonstrate mutual respect.

Self-harm and suicide seem to be related. How will I know my client will not kill themselves?

Voices

Liam

Liam has been in contact with mental health support services for several years. He experienced early onset **psychosis** and was referred to an **Early Intervention Team** and responded well to their support. He was prescribed medication by his psychiatrist and also referred to counselling, where he now sees Andrew. Liam's mental health has deteriorated over recent months, but his psychiatrist still wants to avoid a hospital admission for Liam. Liam has started to take initially small overdoses of his medication, necessitating treatment in A&E.

There is a difficult conundrum to be understood in the relationship between suicide and self-harm, which we have touched on previously. That is, many people who kill themselves have previously self-harmed, but the majority of people who self-harm do not go on to kill themselves. It is too easy to assume a clear relationship between the two, whereas in fact, the relationship is much more complex. It would be wrong therefore, for a counsellor to assume their client is at high risk of suicide simply because they self-harm. However, another important aspect to keep in mind is that self-harm might begin as a mechanism through which people self-support or express difficult feelings but can, over time and following further periods of distress, become life threatening (rather than life sustaining) without the client's awareness.

Liam self-harms through taking small overdoses. Many will interpret an overdose as an attempt to kill oneself, whereas for some an overdose, or ingesting other substances, is in fact an act of self-harm rather than potential suicide. The danger for Liam is that the overdoses over time cause his body irreparable damage, or that the overdoses increase in their frequency or severity so that they become life-threatening, even if Liam does not intend this outcome. It is important for the counsellor, in this case Andrew, to keep this dynamic in mind. It is an important balance to maintain; seeing Liam's behaviour as a form of self-harm but also keeping attentive to the possibility of increased risk.

Andrew's anxieties are likely to be worse if he takes on a position where he tries to 'second guess' Liam's motives or behaviours; interpreting Liam's actions and making assessments accordingly. Rather, Andrew is less likely to feel anxious about this scenario if he is honest with Liam about his speculations and concerns. For example, if Andrew said to Liam, 'You've talked Liam about the overdoses as a form of self-harm. I am also aware of the potential damage they might be causing you so that they become life-threatening over time. I wonder if this is something we can revisit and talk about more?'.

In this dialogue Andrew would help Liam to understand the possible implications of his actions (beyond that of self-harm) and would also be putting risk on the 'agenda' for ongoing or future discussion. This way both Andrew and Liam can work collaboratively in understanding Liam's self-harm and its relation to risk.

If we talk about self-harm will that make matters worse?

Voices

Bonnie

Bonnie is a counsellor working in a voluntary sector agency that offers generic counselling to any adult free of charge. She has been seeing Doreen for several weeks. Doreen is in a violent relationship and feels unable to leave. She been drinking heavily to cope and has alluded to 'other things' she does, without going into detail.

One of the biggest myths about working with suicide risk is that if we ask about the potential for suicide, or about suicidal feelings the client may have, we can increase the risk (Reeves, 2010) – that by naming suicide we can 'put the thought into the client's mind' and that they might be more actively inclined to act on their thoughts. The same myth seems to be present in working with self-harm – that by talking with clients about their self-harm, or by asking clients about self-harm, we might make matters worse.

Bonnie is concerned about Doreen's general well-being and the violence in her relationship at home. She is particularly concerned about the 'other things' Doreen has alluded to but is unsure about whether to ask more, as asking about them might make Doreen do them more, or more severely. However, asking Doreen about the 'other things' in a way in which she has a choice to answer or not is a really important thing to do. First, it communicates to Doreen that what she has said has been heard and is important; second, it communicates that it is okay for Doreen to talk about these things if she chooses to; and third, it opens the way for further discussion about ways in which Doreen self-supports as well as potential risk.

Bonnie might say to Doreen, 'You've talked about "other things" you do Doreen. I wonder if you feel you want to say a little more about that?' Doreen is given the choice whether to talk about these things (as she might not be ready for such a disclosure yet) and, if she is ready, has been given permission by Bonnie to do so. If Doreen declines the offer to talk, that is fine, but Bonnie has at least opened the dialogue about it leaving the way for discussion in the future. Such dialogue, again delivered with empathy and without judgement, can only be a good thing and will not make things worse.

Personal

Deep down I really do not understand it, or 'approve' of it. What can I do?

Voices

Joyce

Joyce is a 34-year-old newly qualified counsellor. During her placement she did not knowingly work with any client who self-harmed. She has recently been referred a new client, Dawn, who has written on her registration form that she 'cut' herself when she felt 'really bad'. Joyce has already noticed a very strong reaction, feeling angry towards Dawn. She simply wants to tell Dawn to 'stop it', but knows she cannot do that.

Our personal responses to self-harm are incredibly important and should not, under any circumstance, be overlooked or pushed away. Even though we may be qualified counsellors, or involved in counsellor training, we are still human (I hope!). We might fear that what we think or feel is not 'right' and might not be approved of by other colleagues. In truth, much of our work with clients is likely to trigger responses, thoughts, feelings and opinions. Clients will tell us much that we might have views about, including suicide, relationships, children, faith and spirituality, the prospect of a termination of pregnancy, alcohol, drugs, violence, or self-harm. It is less important that we have responses to them than it is that we understand what they are, where they come from and how we can 'bracket' them so that we do not act them out in our counselling relationships.

Joyce has had a powerful response to Dawn's disclosure about self-harm, wanting to tell her to 'stop it'. Her response might be informed by a number of factors, including disapproving of self-harm because of faith, feeling incompetent as a counsellor (for the reasons outlined previously), or because of not wanting her client to experience hurt, for example. The factors behind Joyce's response might be many and varied, but the outcome is the same; Joyce has found it difficult to listen to particular aspects of Dawn's story and thus, the counselling relationship is put under threat. It might be that there are important aspects to Joyce's response that could be helpful to the counselling process, if she were able to offer them empathically and without judgement. For example, if Joyce were able to be appropriately **congruent** about her instinctive response to tell Dawn to 'stop' ('When you told me that Dawn I was really aware of wanting to tell you to stop – to protect you somehow'), this might communicate a level of care to Dawn that she had never experienced previously: that someone cared enough about her wellbeing. Obviously Joyce would need to ensure that she reflected on her response, rather than issuing an order!

It would be important for Joyce to explore openly and honestly in supervision how she felt in the session. This highlights the need for the supervision relationship between Joyce and her supervisor to be based on trust and honesty. However, assuming this is the case, the value and importance of supervision in helping counsellors explore their very real and human responses to another's distress is highlighted.

What if I relate to or identify with a client's experience?

Voices

Deshi

Deshi became a counsellor following her own positive experience of therapy. She had struggled with depression and self-harm herself for several years and had attended counselling on the advice of a friend. She knows that counselling is not for everyone, but she still feels that most people could benefit from it, based on her own experience. She has been meeting with Victoria, who experiences depression and also self-harms. Victoria is very hesitant about counselling.

The potential for **identification** with a client, or a client's story, is an ever-present aspect to working as a counsellor. At any given point in counselling, we might be touched by what our clients say, or who they are, and transported into our own experience. The danger here is not the personal identification in itself; it is very likely that all counsellors will, at some point in their career, experience it, but rather how we might respond following such an identification. I also asserted at the beginning of the book that I believe we all self-harm and therefore a 'them' and 'us' distinction between those who do and don't self-harm is unhelpful. We therefore, all have the potential to identify aspects of how our clients self-harm with our own process.

Deshi hears much in Victoria's story that relates to her own, in particular, depression and self-harm. More specifically, Deshi felt greatly helped by her own counselling but is aware of Victoria's uncertainty. The danger here is that Deshi, through a process of identification and previous positive experience, pushes Victoria into counselling when she might not want, or might not be ready for it. The secret in managing anxieties around identification lies in self-awareness; we need to be open to our own responses and consider what they might be about. For Deshi, the temptation to persuade a reluctant or ambivalent Victoria into counselling says much more about Deshi's motivations than Victoria's. Again, the process of supervision is invaluable here. That said, we can only take such considerations to supervision if we are aware of them. Our supervisor might be astute enough to pick up on such dynamics as we talk, but it is better that we as counsellors always reflect on our own motivations and actions so we can respond to clients in a much more informed way.

I do not have a strong stomach: talking in detail about self-harm frightens me

Voices

Sally-Ann

Sally-Ann, a counsellor working in a university setting, works with Adrian, a 19-year-old student who pulls his own hair, picks his skin and picks at scabs. While he is coping academically, Adrian struggles socially and feels very isolated. Sally-Ann experiences Adrian as a warm, compassionate and vulnerable young man, but finds it difficult to hear his accounts of self-harm.

Linked to the previous example of Deshi and Victoria, our responses might also be more visceral than intellectual. It is not uncommon, when working with self-injury or self-harm that is graphically described by clients, or where the injuries are evident, for us to experience strong reactions accordingly. Sally-Ann's experience of Adrian, her client, is almost exclusively positive, so she finds her difficulties in listening to his accounts about his self-harm challenging and she feels badly about herself as a consequence. This is a shame because Sally-Ann's responses are entirely understandable, reasonable and human. They make no comment about her **capacity** to work with Adrian nor her willingness to be his counsellor. Instead, such responses talk of the very real hurt self-harm communicates.

Finding a way of sharing such responses can be extremely helpful. However, great caution is advised here as, without careful consideration, clients can quickly hear judgement and rejection. Such responses cannot be offered to clients without thorough self-reflection and, if possible, careful discussion in supervision. But assuming all these things have taken place, clients can feel that their counsellor is human, 'with them', is warm and that trust can grow.

Sally-Ann might be able to say to Adrian, 'When you describe what you do Adrian, I am very aware of how that impacts on me; how I feel my responses very viscerally and I wonder if that helps me understand what you might feel too?'. Here Sally-Ann has talked of her visceral response without having to name pejorative words that might be experienced as judgemental, instead focusing on her process of response with some suggestion that it might link to Adrian's response. It would not be surprising for Adrian to feel disgusted by his actions and, in hearing Sally-Ann's experience, he might be more willing to share his own thoughts. It is a dialogue to be entered into with care but when offered can be powerfully facilitative.

Is what I can offer going to be enough?

Voices

Clare

Clare is a person-centred counsellor who works with young care-leavers. She thoroughly enjoys her work and feels that counselling offers clients an invaluable space to learn about themselves. She also passionately believes that person-centred counselling is of particular value with this client group as they have had little opportunity to set the direction of their own life. Clare notices, however, that when working with clients who self-harm she doubts the value of her work and often thinks that someone else would be able to help the client more effectively than her.

As has been apparent throughout the case scenarios used here, our personal responses and subsequent anxieties can be powerfully present in our work, especially with clients where self-harm is a feature. None are as insidious as self-doubt, where fears and anxieties about self-harm and our capacity to hear it and work with it in counselling can translate into an inner discourse of not being good enough, or insufficient for our clients. This is subtly different from issues of competence, although confusingly there might sometimes be overlaps.

Clare enjoys her work with this vulnerable client group and feels positively about the work she does but loses her sense of self and value of the counselling specifically around self-harm. It might be that Clare doesn't have the competence to work with self-harm, and she would need to explore this in supervision, but it is more likely that she goes to an anxious place where she loses faith in herself.

Again, supervision would be important here in helping Clare to identify what it is about self-harm that triggers this response and in doing so, identify ways in which she might self-support. There are also parallels here that Clare might additionally wish to explore; how she loses a sense of self during disclosure about self-harm, which might give insight into how her clients lose a sense of themselves during their self-harming process. Such an exploration for Clare might provide powerful insights not only into her own processes and experiences, but those of her clients too.

Summary

As I hope has become apparent in looking at various scenarios and the anxieties we can experience as a consequence, the recurring answers centre on the importance of supervision, self-reflection, honesty and, perhaps most importantly, a willingness to talk and explore with our clients their experience that relates to self-harm. I hope I have demonstrated that with care, empathy, being non-judgemental and a willingness to be open, there are many positives to be gained through dialogue with our clients, not least the alleviation of anxiety.

Further reading

Larcombe, A. (2008) 'Self-Care', in W. Dryden & A. Reeves (eds) *Key Issues for Counselling in Action: Second Edition*. London: Sage, pp. 283–97.

Long, M. & Jenkins, M. (2010) 'Counsellors' perspectives on self-harm and the role of the therapeutic relationship for working with clients who self-harm'. *Counselling and Psychotherapy Research* 10 (3), pp. 192–200.

Chapter 6
Possible impact on clients

The definitions of self-harm offered in earlier chapters of this book tend not to explore the felt experience of people when they self-harm: feelings, thoughts and physical and emotional responses. That is, while definitions set out to clarify what different terms mean, they do not (and perhaps cannot) really give insight into the **process** of self-harm as experienced by the person. It is worth noting here, however, that each individual's experience of their self-harm will be unique to themselves and all we can offer here are insights based on some people's experiences, which may allow us to generalise. It is essential therefore, that you take care and time to explore your client's particular experience so that its meaning is apparent and available for exploration in the counselling process.

The purpose of this chapter is to explore self-harm from a client's inner perspective. That is, the processes that might be at play prior to, during and after self-harm, and more generally from the perspective of someone reflecting on their self-harming experience. I wish to reiterate at this point the position I have taken earlier and throughout this book – that I believe we all self-harm as a means of coping with difficult or stressful events, albeit the extent, nature and severity will differ greatly. This is an important point because it would be easy for this chapter to be about 'those people who self-harm', whereas it is actually about all of us and we all have the opportunity to gain from self-reflection.

I will begin by considering a self-harming process, including triggers to self-harm, its emotional and physiological consequences as well as other aspects people might experience at an **intrapersonal** level (self-esteem, body image), interpersonal level (relationships, intimacy) and a **macro** level (societal perspective, judgements, etc.). All of these aspects will be relevant for counselling and might, either explicitly or implicitly, be explored with your client.

A self-harming process

The process of self-harm I outline in Figure 6.1 is a suggested process that might not necessarily be applicable to every person in every situation. The intention rather is to 'map out' a process that people might go through in building up to their self-harm, and afterwards. The process as outlined might run over a different timescale for each person, or for each situation. For some, this cycle might last for several weeks, for others several hours, while for some others this might be very quick lasting only several minutes. Alternatively, the timescale might be different for each different occasion, so that on one occasion there may be a slow build-up to self-harm over several weeks, but on another occasion for the same person the build-up might only last a few hours or minutes. It is important to help your client understand their particular experience at different times and to explore what aspects might make things different.

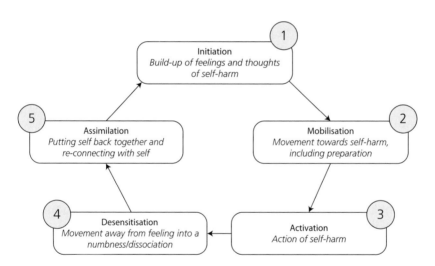

Figure 6.1 A self-harming process

I will outline each stage of Figure 6.1 in a little more detail.

Stage 1: Initiation

During this stage the person will begin to have a sense of building up feelings, or of feelings becoming too difficult to manage or cope with. Such feelings might include anger, frustration, irritation, grief, loss or disgust, for example, and typically are feelings that are difficult to easily express, either because the individual feels immense shame about the feelings or because expression of such feelings is not 'sanctioned' societally. For example, consider Joe's scenario.

Voices

Joe

Joe doesn't really understand why he is so short-tempered but is aware that feelings build up over a period of time and he does not know how to cope with them. He feels angry a great deal of the time but finds that things tend to reach a 'boiling point' before he expresses them, which usually ends up in him getting into trouble.

In Joe's situation he struggles with feelings of anger. Society does not readily sanction anger and, as a consequence, we generally do not know ways to express anger productively or safely. Anger therefore tends to be associated with damage, violence and being out of control. Joe keeps his anger under wraps until a point is reached when it boils over, thus leading to trouble for Joe and further reinforcing the message that anger is a 'bad' feeling. At Stage 1 in Figure 6.1 Joe's feelings of anger might build to the point where he then moves into Stages 2 and 3. However, Joe might be encouraged to find safer ways of expressing his anger as soon as he begins to notice it, thus interrupting the cycle and avoiding anger becoming an aspect of his self-harm.

Stage 2: Mobilisation

Moving on from Stage 1, as the action of self-harm becomes more pressing or immediate there is a sense of being mobilised towards acting on feelings. The can of fizzy drink metaphor can be applied here, where pressure builds to a point of near-explosion in a can of fizzy drink that has been shaken and shaken. Feelings become so intense at Stage 2 that the person is drawn towards the behaviour of self-harm as a means of release or expression of feelings.

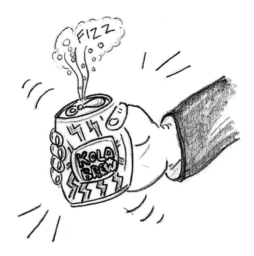

Figure 6.2 Pressure can build like a can of fizzy drink being shaken

Consider Helen's scenario.

Voices

Helen

Helen experienced bullying throughout her school years and she began to cut herself during this time as a means of coping with her feelings. Now at university, the bullying has stopped, but Helen finds that she returns to cutting herself at times of stress. She has a major presentation to do on her course and is highly anxious about it, fearing that she will look stupid and will 'get it wrong'. As the presentation draws near Helen struggles to cope with the escalating feelings of dread. The night before, she cuts herself because she feels so anxious.

Helen's experience is typical of many people who discuss their self-harm in counselling. She began to self-harm during a particularly difficult time in her life in response to her feelings, but even when those initial triggers are no longer present the coping strategy continues unchanged. Helen feels trapped in a cyclical pattern of self-harm, even though she is no longer bullied and generally feels much happier. At Stage 2 of the process Helen does not know how to cope with intense feelings so they become overwhelming. The task in counselling is to help Helen recognise the feelings earlier, much in the same way as we might have done with Joe in the previous scenario, as a means of giving more choices about how she responds to them.

Stage 3: Activation

Following the initiation of feelings and the steady build-up to the point of being overwhelmed, Stage 3 represents the acting out of distress in the form of self-harm. As we have previously discussed, the behaviour of self-harm might include a whole range of actions, from immediate self-injury (cutting, burning), through to deferred self-harm (over-exercise, eating disorders). The point of Stage 3 is that the feelings move into action, and the intensity of response is thus activated. Consider Frederique's scenario.

Voices

Frederique

Frederique has very poor self-esteem and body image. She feels overweight, ugly, too tall and that nobody likes her. She cannot envisage ever having a successful relationship, as she cannot imagine anyone would be attracted to her. For some time Frederique has binge eaten, particularly when she feels disgusted with herself. Recently her closest friend has got into a relationship and this has brought a number of difficult feelings into focus for Frederique. She has been coping with these for several weeks but, having seen photos of her friend with her new partner on Facebook she feels overwhelmed with disgust and begins to binge eat, leading to hating herself even more.

Frederique's experience illustrates the difficult patterns people can easily get caught in around coping with feelings and self-harm. She hates herself and how she looks and binge eats as a means of coping with her self-disgust which, in turn, further adds to her feelings of self-disgust. In this scenario we can easily see Frederique's experience at Stages 1 and 2 of the cycle, with her binge eating representing Stage 3, where she moves from mobilisation into activation, self-harming through her use of food.

Stage 4: Desensitisation

It is not uncommon for people to experience a sense of desensitisation following self-harm, where intense feelings are acted on during the process of harm or injury, which then leads on to a sense of emotional disconnection. The extent of this will depend on the motivation for self-harm, which we will explore shortly, but might include expression of feeling or a need for punishment, for example. After the act of self-harm the person can move into a sense of relief, or shock, which is often typified by a sense of detachment from either themselves or the feelings that triggered the self-harm. For many it is this stage that is the motivation for the self-harm. For example, if feelings are overwhelmingly powerful or difficult to contain or cope with, the thought of being free of them (albeit through a sense of dissociation or disconnection) can be very appealing. The blankness that can be experienced at Stage 4 can feel very soothing in the face of having previously felt overwhelmed (there is a commonality here with the psychological processes that support addiction). Consider Victor's scenario.

Voices

Victor

Victor has been cutting himself for several years. He was sexually assaulted as a child and has never been able to tell anyone about this out of shame and fear of ridicule. He recognises his own process of self-harm, where he begins to feel shame or disgust, which then becomes increasingly powerful, to the point where he cuts himself. Following cutting Victor experiences a period of intense calmness where he feels free from his feelings for a while. This is one of the few times in his life when he feels so calm, and it is this stage he has in his mind when he begins to cut himself.

Victor's sense of calmness is important here in that it is a point at which he feels soothed and calm. The act of cutting himself is a means of releasing powerful feelings but, for Victor, the cutting is not as important as the feelings afterwards. It is worth noting here that some important physiological (as well as psychological) responses are activated. Following injury the body releases endorphins, which are bio-chemicals in the body that act as natural painkillers. They are known to help reduce the sense of pain (like natural opiates) as well as inducing a feeling of well-being or euphoria. It can be very helpful for clients to understand their physiological as well as emotional responses to self-harm as a means of appreciating why they might feel as they do following self-injury. Many people are not aware of the effect of endorphins on the body, nor that endorphins are released following self-harm. Victor's sense of calmness and of being at peace may be as related to his sense of release of feelings as it is to the release of endorphins.

Stage 5: Assimilation

Here I call Stage 5 'assimilation', in that this stage represents a bringing together of a number of factors and of a sense of restoring 'self'. Following Stage 4 and the process of desensitisation, feelings begin to return and the person begins to reconnect with themselves and their world. However, what is important to note is that typically feelings are not experienced in the same intense way as they were at Stage 2; people feel more able to cope again and it is almost as if their feeling intensity has been reset. They are able to function once again and get on with their lives. Consider Eddie's scenario.

Voices

Eddie

Eddie struggles to control his anger. He understands that this relates to a sense of people letting him down, particularly his parents who would neglect him when he was young, leaving him locked in his room for long periods of time. His feelings are triggered now when he feels people overlook him, do not take him seriously or do not do as they promise to do. He manages his anger very privately, however, punching walls and doors when he is on his own. He sometimes causes himself serious injury, including broken bones. Having punched something he then feels calmer and more in control. After a period of time he then feels more able to manage the stresses of day-to-day life, and the process starts over again.

Eddie works hard to function in relationships, even though for a great deal of the time he feels vulnerable and 'bruised' when in them. Intellectually he knows that people typically do not intentionally let him down, unlike his parents, but he is triggered into difficult feelings very quickly. He works hard to function in his relationships and his process of self-harm is, like most peoples', very private. He immediately feels calmer having punched something, finding expression for his anger and frustration, but it is an important 'resetting' process that enables him to move back into relationships again, and not disconnected from them. For Eddie, Stage 5 represents that point at which he is able to almost gather himself together, ground himself and reconnect with his life.

Activity

Take the stages as outlined in Figure 6.2 and consider a client you are currently working with. Reflect on how the stages might help provide insight into their process. You might do this on your own, or with your supervisor. Alternatively, think of yourself and how you cope with particular stresses or difficulties and see if the stages throw any light onto your own experience of coping.

Why we self-harm and its consequences

We self-harm for a variety of reasons that differ for each individual and situation. While there are broad explanations for self-harm, it is important that we offer clients space and time to consider what is relevant for them, and how that might vary from situation to situation. Particular triggers to self-harm can include:

- self-hatred
- self-punishment
- stress
- guilt
- loss of control
- sense of isolation
- grief
- to feel something
- for a sense of relief
- to purge
- anger
- despair
- low self-esteem.

As we can see, the list could be almost limitless and will essentially relate to the client's particular experiences or problems. For some people self-harm might be about seeking a sense of relief from overwhelming feelings, or might be in response to high levels of anger, despair or grief. For others, however, self-harm might be to experience pain, where the status quo is more about disconnection from self and living in an anaesthetised state. When we **dissociate** from strong or powerful feelings we can almost forget that we feel at all; self-harm in that context can be very affirming in demonstrating that feeling is possible at all. The consequences of self-harm, as we have already outlined in the scenarios above, can be experienced at an emotional/psychological level and at a physiological level. Emotionally we might experience:

- a sense of relief
- a sense of being purged from something disgusting
- a feeling of regaining control
- distracting ourselves from the deeper hurt
- a confirmation of our existence
- creating a focus for the hurt (where it is otherwise felt generally and overwhelmingly).

Whereas physiologically we might experience:

- a release of endorphins
- a dulling of the immediate sense of pain
- lifting of mood
- greater sense of euphoria or well-being
- sense of physical calmness and peace.

There can be an important role for psycho-education when working with self-harm. It is not uncommon for people to fear their self-harm is a sign of serious mental health problems, or that no one would understand how or why they do it. To be able to explain some of the above can be immensely supporting and affirming, creating opportunities for further exploration in a non-judgemental and supportive way. For example, for people to understand the process and meaning of their self-harm can be quite powerful in helping them to talk about things that might otherwise sit beyond their **capacity** to do so. This is called psycho-education, where we offer information and explanation rooted in the context of the individual's particular experience of themselves or their situation.

Other consequences of self-harm

I have outlined above the immediate consequences of self-harm, but there may be others too that can be described as **intrapersonal** consequences, interpersonal consequences and **macro** consequences. I will consider each in turn.

Intrapersonal consequences

Intrapersonal ('taking place or existing within the mind', Oxford Dictionaries, 2013) relates to those factors to do with our relationship with ourselves; that is, how self-harm influences our view of our self and how that can be shaped by what we do. My own experience of working with self-harm in counselling is that how self-harm informs a client's view of themselves can be as profound as, or often more so, than the actual act of self-harm itself. As we have discussed in earlier chapters, the temptation for counsellors is to focus on the actual behaviour of self-harm, usually in an attempt to reduce it (perhaps to make us feel better?). However, what is often more relevant to the client is how they *feel* about the self-harm in relation to themselves.

It is not uncommon for people to make very harsh judgements about themselves because of their self-harm. They get caught in a vicious cycle, where self-harm (as a means of coping with difficult feelings) begins to create difficult feelings because of the sense of shame or self-judgement they feel. Self-harm then occurs not only because of the original triggers, but because the client self-harms as a means of coping with these additional feelings. Consider Shane's scenario.

Voices

Shane

Shane feels worthless because of sexual abuse he experienced when he was younger. As a means of coping with his sense of low self-esteem and other feelings, such as anger, disgust and shame, he cuts himself on his legs (where no one can see). He hates himself for this behaviour as he thinks he should be coping better and should be 'stronger': he feels he is also a weak person for cutting himself. These add to his pre-existing feelings of anger, disgust and shame and he continues to cut himself also as a punishment for being so 'weak and pathetic'.

Likewise, the impact on a client's body of self-harm can additionally add to feelings of low self-esteem by adding in reduced or poor body image. Again, reflecting on Shane's experience:

Voices

Shane (continued)

Shane further struggles to cope with the scars on his legs and feels that no one will ever find him attractive. He cannot bear the thought of people seeing what he considers to be his weakness scarred on his body, so he withdraws from the potential of relationships. He feels badly about his body, badly about himself and increasingly trapped in his own separate and shameful world.

As we can see, the intrapersonal consequences of self-harm can be profound for people and often can trap them in a way of being that centres around their self-harm. Counselling can provide an important space for these intrapersonal dynamics to be discussed and explored and, perhaps most importantly, sensitively brought into the open to help break what might otherwise be a cyclic self-reinforcing process.

Interpersonal consequences

Interpersonal ('relating to relationships or communication between people', Oxford Dictionaries, 2013) refers to how relationships with others can be shaped and informed by the process of self-harm. For most people, despite the assumptions often made to the contrary, self-harm is a very private intrapersonal process. It is something we keep to ourselves because we struggle with what we do, or fear that others will judge us. It is not uncommon for self-harm to have a profound impact on a person's confidence to begin new relationships, or develop existing relationships. This impact can be felt around:

- emotional intimacy, where the fear is of letting other people in to a self-harming process, or at a
- **relational** level, where people might struggle with issues of trust and sharing, or at a
- sexual level, where sexual intimacy is feared for fear of judgement, particularly when the self-harm causes physical injury.

Let us revisit Shane's situation.

Voices

Shane (continued)

Shane's partner, Davy, feels that Shane is quite withdrawn from him, reluctant to go out, reluctant to spend time with friends, questioning and challenging of day-to-day things and, increasingly, reluctant to have sex. He and Shane have been in a relationship for 18 months but Davy feels that he is never allowed to be close to Shane and that he still, after this time, does not really know him. He feels shut out of Shane's world and does not know how to make the connection.

While Shane is desperate for relationships and relational intimacy, he fears the consequences of letting Davy share his thoughts and feelings. He fears Davy's judgement of him for his actions, or repulsion at his body. Relationships feel risky and the more Shane feels Davy's frustration at the current situation, the less he feels able to take those risks. Again, here we see a cyclical process that can quickly trap the person and their partner (and friends and family). Similarly to the intrapersonal consequences, counselling can provide a safe space for the client to begin to explore how their self-harm shapes and influences their relationships with others and to consider ways in which they might begin to make changes to allow greater levels of intimacy and closeness.

Macro consequences

Macro ('large-scale, overall', Oxford Dictionaries, 2013) relates to those aspects that transcend the individual and relational and are more to do with the societal perspective of self-harm that can be internalised by the individual. As outlined earlier, it is not uncommon for people to come into counselling with a range of pre-conceptions about self-harm and what that might say about them: they are weak; they are weird; they cannot cope; they are mentally ill; they should be 'locked up'; they are dangerous; they are suicidal, and so on. It is probably fair to say that in a Western culture there is little understanding or tolerance of self-harm, where instead the predominant discourse is of coping, normal (whatever that is), in control, successful, aspirational, and so on. For the final time, let us revisit Shane.

Voices

Shane (continued)

In counselling Shane talks about how weak he feels and how he thinks he should cope better. He struggles to name his feelings, instead taking a clear intellectual position about himself that is devoid of feeling or empathy. He is very self-critical and self-judgemental. He grew up in a family with a very dominant father, where being male was about being stoic, in control and not expressing emotions. For Shane, his self-harm is an affront to his perceived sense of what it is to be a man.

As we can see, our views of ourselves will be shaped by the societal context in which we live. As such, issues of age, gender, sexuality, ability or disability and culture will be profound influencing factors in our position in relation to self-harm. It is important that, as counsellors, we take into account these wider contextual factors and therefore be **systemic** in our thinking. That is, we must consider the systems in which people live and function as well as focusing on their individual **narrative**. In the example of Shane, his socialisation as a male in a society that privileges masculinity as dominant, powerful and in control is a powerful factor in **intra-** and **interpersonal** perspectives.

Intervention strategies

Let us briefly revisit Figure 6.1, but instead consider how we might support clients to make changes, as illustrated in Figure 6.3.

At Stage 1 (initiation), we can help clients think about what factors, experiences or issues might arise in their day-to-day lives that might trigger the pull towards self-harm. If clients are able to identify these early on then they are better positioned to find alternative mechanisms for self-support.

At Stage 2 (mobilisation) it can be helpful to work with clients on increased self-awareness; not just cognitively, but also emotionally and physically. Sometimes it is possible to recognise an increase in tension and take steps to reduce anxiety or frustration through the use of breathing techniques, relaxation techniques or mindfulness, for example.

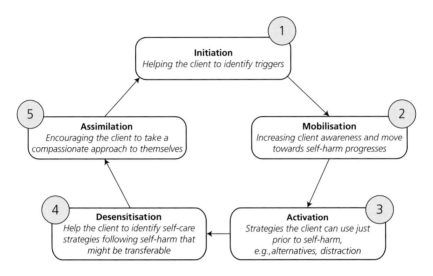

Figure 6.3 Intervention options

At Stage 3 (activation) the client may be able to make use of alternatives to self-harm that have been developed over time by people who have found them useful. The Royal College of Psychiatrists produce an excellent document you can print out and give to clients, discussing with them strategies they might be drawn to. The link for this document is at the end of this chapter in 'Further reading'.

Stage 4 (desensitisation) is a point at which a client may move towards self-care, particularly focusing on any injuries they might have sustained. As we saw in Chapter 3 with Zac, this can also prove to be a positive point of change.

Finally, Stage 5 (assimilation) is a point where the client may feel profoundly guilty or ashamed of their actions. Encouraging a more self-compassionate and forgiving approach can begin to help the client see themselves from a different position which, in turn, might be used at different stages of the cycle.

Summary

In summary, we have considered a process of self-harm that follows a person's experience from the earliest stages of self-harm through to post-self-harm consequences, including factors that will be experienced at an intra- and interpersonal level, as well as wider factors. All of these are, of course, generalisations and cannot do justice to each individual's account of their own experience and the particular sense that they make of it. Here counselling has an important role in opening up what might otherwise be closed and self-reinforcing processes, which has the potential to help clients find alternative ways of being.

Further reading

Babiker, G. & Arnold, L. (1997) *The Language of Injury: Comprehending Self-Mutilation*. Oxford: Wiley-Blackwell.

Royal College of Psychiatrists (2013) *Alternatives to Self-Harm and Distraction Techniques*. **www.rcpsych.ac.uk/PDF/Self-Harm Distractions and Alternatives FINAL.pdf** (accessed 17 December 2012).

Turp, M. (1999) 'Encountering self-harm in psychotherapy and counselling practice'. *British Journal of Psychotherapy* 15 (3), pp. 306–21.

Chapter 7
Professional issues

Thinking beyond the relationship

As a counsellor working in any setting, and with any presenting issue, there are a number of important professional considerations that must be fully attended to in ensuring the best possible level of care for clients. People who seek out, or are referred for, counselling are often at their most vulnerable with high levels of distress. They are highly dependent on you, the counsellor, to ensure that every step has been taken to offer a safe, respectful and ethical working context. Only in such a context should counselling take place, for without such consideration the danger of harm to the client (and indeed to the counsellor) can be high.

As we have discussed already, clients may present in counselling with a specific goal to work on of reducing their self-harming behaviour, or instead might not want to particularly focus on self-harm. Instead they might see it as a representation of their struggle, rather focusing on the causes of the distress and difficulty themselves. In that sense self-harm differs slightly from some other client presentations. For example, a client may attend counselling following bereavement or a trauma, to discuss their experience. It may be that self-harm is also a feature for them, but it may not be. I have cautioned in previous chapters against being self-harm-focused (unless it is the goal of the client to look specifically at self-harm), instead to allow for the client to set the agenda for counselling.

With this in mind it is important to remember that, for many clients, self-harm is an aspect of their distress, but often not the source of the distress itself: self-harm is an expression (or sometimes acting-out) of hurt, rather than the hurt itself. This is illustrated in Figure 7.1. As you can see, I suggest three significant points:

1. the self-harm that is visible to others
2. the way in which self-harm is related to its cause (the source of the distress)
3. the impact of self-harm on the client (for example, self-esteem, body image, etc.)

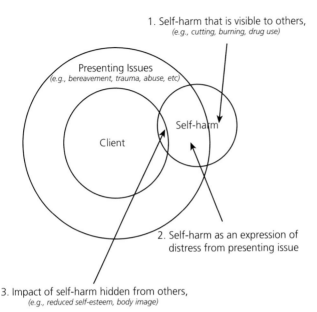

Figure 7.1 Locating self-harm in the context of client distress

How we might work therapeutically with each of these areas has already been discussed in Chapter 3. At this point, however, Figure 7.1 serves simply to illustrate that, as counsellors, we can too quickly become focused on point 1, without paying sufficient attention to points 2 and 3. This contextualises the importance of us paying careful attention to a range of professional considerations that sit within, but also beyond the therapeutic relationship itself.

Key professional considerations

So, what are the key professional considerations that we must keep in mind in our work with clients, and with clients where self-harm is also a presenting factor? I would group them into two main categories: relationship-based considerations; and role-based considerations. To explain further, relationship-based considerations are those that relate to our direct work with clients and that sit beyond the more extensive considerations related to therapeutic skills and techniques. Whereas role-based considerations are those related to our work as counsellors in the wider frame. Below I have listed some considerations that I will look at further in this chapter.

- **Relationship-based considerations**
  - Contracting
  - Maintaining the focus of counselling
  - Reviewing
  - Use of Supervision
  - Self-care
- **Role-based considerations**
  - Working ethically
  - Employment and working context
  - Continuing professional development
  - Accreditation and registration
  - Disagreements and complaints

Relationship-based considerations

Contracting

Contracting is an important aspect of all counselling and should not be rushed or made simply into a routine task. The danger is that we talk through the aspects of the contract, including confidentiality, quite quickly because we are so familiar with it ourselves. However, it is important to keep in mind that for many people this will be their first experience of counselling and the language we are so familiar with will not necessarily be as clear or apparent to our clients, who may at the same time be experiencing high levels of distress or vulnerability. Consider Maureen's scenario.

Voices

Maureen

Maureen has never been to counselling previously but it has been recommended to her by a close friend. She has confided in her friend that, following the breakdown of a long-term relationship, she has started to cut herself. Maureen goes to see a counsellor, who she experiences as very warm and welcoming. The counsellor seems to be open, honest and willing to listen to Maureen's difficulties. The counsellor explains a number of things in the first session, about fees, frequency, cancellation and, at one point, says that things will be confidential unless she is concerned about Maureen's 'safety or the safety of others', in which case she might speak to Maureen's GP. Maureen does not really know what this means and is too anxious to ask. However, she concludes that it would probably be best not to talk about her self-harm for fear that her GP will find out and it will be recorded on her medical notes.

Activity

Think about Maureen's scenario and reflect on the following questions:

- How might the counsellor have checked with Maureen her understanding of the contract?
- How could the counsellor introduce and talk about the contract differently?
- What do you recognise in your own practice from the scenario in relation to contracting? What changes, if any, might you make?

In this scenario we see Maureen taking an important (and frightening) step in seeking out counselling for the first time. Her counsellor is warm and welcoming and sets out to contract so that Maureen understands the terms of the counselling. Maureen struggles with this because: a) she is anxious about seeing a counsellor for the first time; b) is distressed about the breakdown of her relationship; c) feels ashamed about cutting herself and worried about telling someone else, particularly a stranger; d) is given a lot of information to remember in a short period of time; and e) is not entirely clear about some of the language the counsellor uses. She decides it is better to keep the information about her self-harm to herself: the counsellor has intended to create a warm and safe environment for Maureen but has, in fact, silenced her. The importance of taking time over contracting, having it written down (or presented in a form that is accessible and understandable to the client, such as braille or audio-recorded), clearly explaining terms and, most importantly, clearly outlining exactly what is meant by the limitations to confidentiality, will best provide for a relationship in which the client can trust and talk about difficult things.

Maintaining the focus of counselling

I make no apologies for returning so often to the point about not becoming self-harm focused during counselling because it is a trap that so many of us can quickly fall into. Our openness to hearing the client's full **narrative** can quickly disappear once self-harm comes into the frame. Consider Christine's scenario.

Voices

Christine

Christine goes to her first counselling session and is invited by her counsellor to talk about what is worrying her. She tells her counsellor a number of things, including her experience of sexual abuse when she was younger, difficulties in ongoing relationships now, periods of anger and upset, poor self-esteem and poor body image. The counsellor invites Christine to consider where she would like to begin and what she would like the focus of early sessions to be. On reflection, Christine says the ongoing relationship issues, which they begin to discuss. During the third session Christine decides to **disclose** to her counsellor that she has, for many years, burnt herself with cigarettes on her arms, particularly when feeling very angry. While the counsellor seems accepting of this information, Christine becomes frustrated with an increasing focus on her self-harm during subsequent sessions, but does not feel able to tell her counsellor this.

Activity

Think about Christine's scenario and reflect on the following questions:
- Is the counsellor right to focus more on the self-harm, given that Christine introduced it into the session?
- Presumably Christine wanted to talk about her self-harm, given the fact that she told her counsellor. Would you agree?
- How might the counsellor have responded differently to Christine's disclosure?

The counsellor took great care to ensure that Christine remained in control of the focus of counselling and took time to facilitate Christine thinking about the areas of her life she felt to be of most immediate need. It would have been easy for the counsellor to assume that Christine's experience of abuse was the core of her problems and, as such, would have been the natural start. But the counsellor recognised that while this was possibly true, Christine might not have been able to begin with such traumatic experiences so early on in the counselling. As Christine began to trust her counsellor she felt able to talk a little more about the different ways in which her distress impacted on her, including burning herself. However, the counsellor, while appearing to be able to hear this information, instead reacted strongly and allowed her own anxiety to begin to set the focus for counselling without checking this out with Christine. The importance of ensuring the client's focus remains central is illustrated here. While it would have been valuable for the counsellor to check issues of risk with Christine, a better response might simply have been to have asked Christine, 'That seems important for you to have told me that. Is that something you would like to focus on now, or would you prefer we continue with the areas we have already been discussing?'

Reviewing

Having worked through the contract and helped your client set the focus of counselling, it is important to set time aside with your client to check whether the original focus is still correct, or whether things have changed. Like most things in life, the passage of time will often bring about change in itself and the same is true for counselling. If working briefly of course, there is less time for reviewing as sessions are time-limited. However, time-limited counselling might be eight to ten sessions, which would still allow for a period of review. The purpose of reviewing counselling is to provide you and your client with an opportunity to reflect on what, if anything, is different and how changes might require a different focus for the work. Failure to review counselling while it is in progress can lead to stagnant and unhelpful work, where the client feels trapped in a **process** they might not feel able to challenge or change. Consider Duncan's scenario.

Voices

Duncan

Duncan has been seeing his counsellor for three months. When he began counselling he was asked by his counsellor to consider the focus for the work. Duncan said that his major concern was his dangerous and 'reckless' behaviour, (for example, sleeping around, fast driving, taking risks with his health) and this became the focus. As the counselling has progressed Duncan has become increasingly aware of just how badly he feels about himself and how that stems from being in local authority care when he was younger. While he has named this with his counsellor, the counselling has continued to focus on Duncan's behaviours rather than his feelings about himself. He does not want to talk about how frustrated he is because: a) he likes his counsellor and does not want to upset him; and b) he feels his needs have always been overlooked and this is just another example.

Activity

Think about Duncan's scenario and reflect on the following questions:
- Why might Duncan's counsellor continue to focus on his behaviours rather than the feelings about himself Duncan is beginning to describe?
- How might the counsellor go about reviewing the counselling, and why?
- If the counselling was reviewed, what might be different for Duncan?

The danger in all counselling when we do not review is that we continue to address problems that have been resolved or, over time, have simply gone away. We can inadvertently leave our clients feeling stuck. This is particularly true if the focus is self-harm because of our anxiety for it to 'get better', as we have discussed previously. The value of reviewing, therefore, is to provide a discrete space in which we can ask the client whether the counselling continues to be helpful, what, if anything, might have changed and whether new areas have emerged for us to consider instead.

Use of supervision

In the UK supervision is a requirement of good practice. It is not a **statutory** requirement, but one instead that is based in ethics and values. As counsellors we are required to meet regularly with an experienced practitioner (a supervisor) to discuss our work with clients and ourselves as practitioners. Supervision provides us with a space to consider the quality of our work (normative factors), the nature of our work and ways of working (formative factors), as well as considering the impact of our work on ourselves (restorative factors) (Inskipp & Proctor, 1993). Its importance in working with self-harm becomes quickly apparent when considering the three primary functions of supervision as outlined here. Consider Andreas' scenario.

Voices

Andreas

Andreas has been working with Stuart for several weeks. Stuart gets into fights but also cuts himself. He has a very poor relationship with his parents, particularly his father, whom he blames for much of his distress. His father was violent towards both Stuart's mother and Stuart himself. Stuart feels worthless a lot of the time, but angry too. Andreas often feels verbally 'attacked' by Stuart and the focus of his anger (although does not feel physically threatened). He is not really sure how to respond for fear of further aggravating Stuart's anger.

Activity

Think about Andreas' scenario and reflect on the following questions:
- What do you consider to be the important links between Stuart's experiences when growing up and his current problems?
- What might be the reasons for how Andreas feels in his work with Stuart?
- What might Andreas need to do to find a way forward?

Andreas felt a little ashamed about talking with his supervisor about his work with Stuart, because he felt he should be doing better and should not be so anxious about his client's responses to him. However, when he did he found it of enormous benefit. The supervisor helped Andreas to consider the levels of risk in the relationship and whether he and Stuart were both safe (normative considerations). The supervisor also paid close attention to how Andreas had been feeling and the potential costs to him as a counsellor, but also to the work with Stuart. It became apparent that Andreas had been 'backing off' from the relationship, not offering thoughts or responses, and that the relationship had suffered because of it. Andreas found it immensely helpful to have named these dynamics and for the supervisor to understand – he felt less ashamed about what had been going on (restorative considerations).

Finally, the supervisor had helped Andreas think more deeply about what might be going on between him and Stuart, including the possibility of **transferential** dynamics (where Stuart was responding to Andreas as a male authority figure who became representative of his father) and the importance of finding a way of exploring this with Stuart (formative considerations). The value of supervision is very clear in this example and shows in all our work as counsellors, and particularly when working with self-harming **processes**, the importance of the supervisory frame for support and insight.

Self-care

Self-care is an ethical requirement of good practice. However, it may be fair to say that while many counsellors would entirely endorse the principle of self-care, it is an aspect of practice that can quickly be overlooked amidst the demands of day-to-day work. We have already discussed the emotional and physical demands working with self-harm can place on the counsellor. The danger of vicarious trauma, as previously defined, is very real when we manage our empathic responses following disclosures of self-harm. Also, the demands on counselling services often result in counsellors working long hours, with many clients, with little regard possible for the demands the work makes on the individual practitioner. Consider Victoria's scenario.

Voices

Victoria

Victoria works in a third-sector agency working with young women. She works full-time and sees five, sometimes six clients every day. Given the nature of her agency many of her clients talk about their self-harm, which Victoria sometimes finds difficult, and other times feels 'cut off' from. With her partner she has two young children and finds that her time away from work is taken up with caring for her children. When she gives herself time to think, Victoria feels angry and frustrated that she spends so much of her life looking after everyone else and so little time looking after herself. She feels tired most of the time and emotionally and physically drained.

Activity

Think about Victoria's scenario and reflect on the following questions:
- Why might Victoria be angry and frustrated and how might that relate to her client work?
- What might the costs be for: a) Victoria; and b) her clients, of this situation continuing?
- What could Victoria do?

Here we can see an obvious parallel between how Victoria works with self-harm and how then Victoria begins to do things that might also be self-harming. For example, in her direct work with clients Victoria can sometimes experience difficult emotions, while at other times **dissociate** so that she 'cuts off' her feelings, in much the same way as her clients might. The cost for Victoria is that she feels overwhelmed, drained and emotionally exhausted – her mental and physical health are in jeopardy, her **capacity** to be with clients can become impaired, she begins to struggle caring for her children and her relationship with her partner suffers. All in all, the costs are high. The reality is that there may be some aspects Victoria does not have the power to change (for example, her clients will continue to bring difficult and challenging **narratives** into counselling). However, there may be other aspects of her life that Victoria assumes she cannot change, but might be able to, and still other things she can definitely change.

Supervision is again important here in helping Victoria think about the impact of her work on herself and achieve some clarity about what she might be able to do. This might include:

- discussing with her line manager a system of caseload management that takes into account the demands of working with risk
- ensuring she takes whatever time is available at work for recovery, (such as taking a walk out of the office at lunchtime to take herself away from the work environment)
- discussing with her partner childcare demands and how they might work between them
- building in some time for exercise
- building in some time for other restorative activities, (such as taking a bath, reading, listening to music, eating well)
- discussing with her supervisor the process of developing a self-care plan.

These are simply ideas and you might identify a number of other, and different, things you could do for yourself. It is important to reflect on all aspects of our professional and personal needs. Larcombe (2008, p. 290–3) outlines the need to care for our *therapeutic self, managerial self* and *career self*. The therapeutic self is the part related to the impact on ourselves of our work with clients. The managerial self includes workload, deadlines, working environment and professional relationships, for example, while the career self relates to making links between our current work and how we envisage our role developing in the future. Attending to all these areas in a coherent plan that we can review can work towards protecting our own well-being and to ensuring we remain as psychologically available to clients as possible.

Role-based considerations
Working ethically

Membership of a professional organisation in the UK, and typically internationally too, requires adherence to an ethical framework or code of ethics. Such a framework sets clear benchmarks for what is considered to be safe and respectful practice, which are based not only on parameters of what we should and should not 'do', but also on principles, philosophical aspects and values that underpin the very nature of counselling. I will discuss ethical aspects of working with self-harm in counselling in much more detail in Chapter 8. Here, however, the intention is simply to locate ethical practice and ethical thinking as an important professional requirement. Consider Jordan's scenario.

Voices

Jordan

Jordan is a counsellor who works with Betty, a cardiologist. Betty has approached Jordan, an independent practitioner, as she did not want to access counselling through her own GP due to anxiety about concerns being expressed regarding her fitness to practise medicine. Betty has struggled with anxiety, panic attacks and negative intrusive thoughts for many years. When things are particularly difficult she drinks heavily and has, on occasion, cut herself. She feels very ashamed of her drinking and particularly her cutting. She is fearful that, if found out, she might be 'struck off' from practice. Jordan is anxious about Betty's capacity to support herself and, as a consequence, provide a safe service for her patients. However, he is also very reluctant to break Betty's confidentiality as he also recognises the important step she has taken in coming to counselling as a mechanism of self-support and possible change.

Activity

Think about Jordan's scenario and reflect on the following questions:
- What are the primary ethical considerations for Jordan?
- In your view what is the balance of harm to Betty's patients verses harm to Betty if she is 'struck off' or does not feel able to come to counselling any more?
- What would you do in such a situation, and how would you reach that conclusion?

Whatever Jordan decides to do, and however he reaches this decision (using supervision and in dialogue with Betty herself), he has to embed his thinking in ethics. While harm to Betty's patients is at the forefront of his mind, he is also aware of the enormous step Betty has taken in recognising the problems she faces and seeking out help of her own volition. The danger is that if Jordan raises his concerns with a third party (with or without Betty's consent) he runs the risk of undermining Betty's trust in the security of counselling and thus undermines it as a source of potential support and change for Betty. We often think of ethics only when we hit particular boundary issues and look for them to show us a 'right' or 'wrong' way.

Instead, it is preferable for us to engage in an ongoing process of ethical thinking so that, at any given stage, we can locate our practice accordingly within safe parameters. In this scenario it is my view, on balance, that Jordan should discuss his concerns with Betty in the context of undertaking an assessment of risk, so that she is aware of his thinking, but that he should respect her confidentiality. Further concern might be raised if, as the sessions continue, Betty cannot seem to change her situation or things deteriorate. At that point Jordan might revisit the discussion with Betty to agree a way forward keeping in mind both her own well-being but that of her patients.

Employment and working context

We have discussed in Chapter 2 how the working context can shape the nature of the counselling being offered and how self-harm can further shape that frame. The important consideration here is an acknowledgement that the nature of our employment and working context will inform some of the way we might work with self-harm. For example, we might have less freedom to dictate our own policies and working practices if based within a health care setting than if we were working independently. Consider Sammy's scenario.

Voices

Sammy

Sammy is a counsellor who works in two settings. For three days per week she works in a primary care counselling agency seeing clients referred by their GP. The organisation has a clear policy that all **disclosures** of self-harm should be reported back to the referring GP for additional assessment. This is made clear to clients at referral. Two days per week Sammy runs her own independent practice seeing clients who make direct contact with her. Sammy's own working practice is that self-harm remains confidential, unless she suspects that it is becoming so severe or chaotic that it is becoming life-threatening.

Activity

Think about Sammy's scenario and reflect on the following questions:
- What are your own particular responses to these two approaches to working with risk? Why do you think they are so different?
- Which policy are you more inclined to agree with, and why?
- What might be the challenges for Sammy in managing these two very different ways of working?

There can be challenges for counsellors when working in a setting where the expectations of practice are not congruent with personally held views (Reeves & Mintz, 2001). Sammy sets her own preferred working practices when working independently, but in the health care setting has to work within the parameters set by the organisation, even if she personally disagrees with them. It may be that she is able to challenge them and open up discussion about their professional or ethical viability, but if she was unsuccessful in changing the policy she would still have to subscribe to it as an employee of the organisation bound by the terms of her working contract. What is important here is that Sammy does not simply ignore the policy because she doesn't agree with it.

The danger is that when we disagree with something we do our own thing anyway. This is unhelpful because it leaves us exposed should things go wrong, and also unhelpful to our clients who begin therapy with an understanding of the parameters that then change without warning: a bit like contracting for a 50-minute session only to let the session go on for an hour and a half. Clear parameters help set the therapeutic frame which in turn contributes to the safety of the working environment and therapeutic relationship.

Continuing professional development

Continuing professional development (CPD) is, for many professional organisations, an ethical requirement for membership and future registration. This is not just in counselling and psychotherapy, but other professions too, such as social work, nursing, teaching and psychology. Gaining our initial qualification is essential in ensuring we have sufficient knowledge and competency to deliver counselling safely and appropriately. However, as the old adage goes, once we pass our driving test we then really begin to learn how to drive. This is very true for counselling where, on qualification, we should be able to do what is necessary to establish, sustain and successfully end therapeutic relationships. However, many aspects of our work will demand further knowledge and/or self-reflection, and this is very true for working with self-harm. Consider Alexander's scenario.

Voices

Alexander

Alexander has recently qualified and secured a job as a part-time counsellor. His placement had been well-organised and managed and all clients were assessed for suitability for a trainee prior to him seeing them. In his new setting he has already met a couple of clients for whom self-harm is a presenting factor. He feels anxious about this and is very aware of feeling out of his depth: not really understanding why people might harm themselves. He is advised by his supervisor to seek out and attend a workshop or training to help equip him in his work.

Activity

Think about Alexander's scenario and reflect on the following questions:
- What are your thoughts about the placement's policy of always assessing clients for their suitability for a trainee in preparing Alexander for the realities of practice?
- Should Alexander now be working with self-harm and how might he do that safely?
- What should his next steps be?

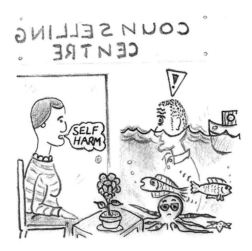

Figure 7.2 The counsellor might feel out of their depth

The supervisor's suggestion for Alexander to seek out CPD to help equip him to work with issues of self-harm has normative (ensuring the safety and appropriateness of the counselling), restorative (paying attention to Alexander's needs and anxieties), and formative (signposting Alexander to acquire new knowledge and skills) aspects. There are some excellent CPD opportunities available to provide space and time to develop knowledge, skills and confidence to work more effectively with self-harm, and these should be taken by both newly qualified and experienced counsellors. Affirming existing skills can be as important as developing new ones, as can challenging long-held beliefs or assumptions that do not fully reflect the nature of the work being undertaken.

Accreditation and registration

For several years in the UK the government agenda was for the statutory regulation of counselling and psychotherapy. That is, people would not be able to practise as counsellors or psychotherapists without meeting national benchmarks of qualification and competence and being registered. A change in the UK government led to a change in priorities, and plans for statutory regulation were dropped. At the time of writing, a plan for the implementation of voluntary registers, held and maintained through professional networks, is underway and it is anticipated that as many counsellors as possible will be encouraged to sign up for one of the registers. Alongside this sits professional accreditation: counsellors applying to a professional organisation to become accredited members, having to demonstrate a number of competencies and meet benchmarked training standards. These initiatives are aimed at raising the professional standards in counselling and at helping make the profession more accountable for its practice. Consider Desmond's scenario.

Voices

Desmond

Desmond has been qualified for two years and works as a voluntary counsellor. He has been trying to find paid employment but most jobs require applicants to be accredited with a professional organisation. Desmond, therefore, does not meet essential criteria for many jobs but feels that in his work he has gained a great deal of client experience, particularly around self-harm, which he would like to be recognised.

Activity

Think about Desmond's scenario and reflect on the following questions:
- What do you think are the relative costs and benefits of accreditation?
- Do you think working with particular client groups (for example, with self-harm) should have specific recognition or is generic accreditation sufficient?
- What should Desmond do next to develop his career?

While there are CPD opportunities to acquire and develop skills around working with self-harm, accreditation, as it stands, is not linked to working within any particular specialism. For some organisations this is in a process of change where accreditation can be linked to particular settings and clients groups (for example, children and young people). However, while working with self-harm is not, as yet, seen as a particular area of competency for accreditation or registration, such experience is invaluable in demonstrating ethical thinking and professional standards. It would be important to highlight this area of experience in your application, closely linking it to any ethical frameworks you are required to subscribe to as part of your membership.

Disagreements and complaints

Most professional organisations that represent counselling have a process for complaint. Some interesting research has audited complaints received, showing that in relation to the wide availability of counselling and the probability of the vast number of sessions delivered per year nationally, relatively few complaints are made (Khele *et al*, 2008; Symons *et al*, 2011; Symons 2012). Major transgressions or abuse of clients need to be formally and properly investigated by counselling or professional organisations.

However, short of serious malpractice, such as the abuse of clients, there may be a number of factors that contribute to problems or difficulties, (boundary issues, fees, miscommunication or failure to communicate, for example). It might be asserted that for a problem to reach a formal complaint in itself represents a failure to address issues properly and in communication. The task for all counsellors is to respond as fully and openly as possible when it transpires that problems have arisen, in an attempt to find a satisfactory resolution. By its very nature counselling focuses on very personal aspects of human experience and the need to carefully respect people's experience is great. Consider Emile's scenario.

Voices

Emile

Emile has been working with Antony for several weeks, looking at issues to do with trauma and loss, as well as cutting and burning himself. Emile has been deliberately tentative in her interventions with Antony, recognising his vulnerability and how quickly he hears criticism. During a session she makes a suggested link between his self-harming and a particular experience he has had. Antony hears this as criticism, becomes upset and walks out of the session. Emile contacts him later by email (as previously agreed at the contract as the best means of contacting him) and invites him to a session to talk about what has happened.

Activity

Think about Emile's scenario and reflect on the following questions:
- What are your thoughts about how tentative Emile has been with Antony, and how she might have worked with this differently?
- Do you see what has happened as an irretrievable fracture in the relationship?
- How might Emile manage the next session?

If this situation is not responded to quickly, with care and empathy, the danger is that harm occurs and the relationship is lost. Emile loses confidence in herself as a therapist and in the value of her interventions, while Antony feels criticised and worse about himself, perhaps not returning to counselling in the future. This scenario demonstrates the need for us to be honest with our clients about how we work and the types of interventions we might make, as well as responding with the same level of honesty and empathy in the face of difficulties. It is important to recognise the high levels of shame clients may experience in coming to counselling at all, and more so if their **narrative** includes aspects of self-harm.

Summary

We have outlined here a number of important professional considerations that are essential in working with self-harm, as well as more general practice. Taking these considerations into account can help to ensure we offer the best possible setting for our clients, as well as engaging with our personal and professional development as an ongoing process. The relationship-focused and role-focused considerations here highlight how professional development sits in the therapeutic relationship, but also beyond it too.

Further reading

Reeves, A. & Howdin, J. (2010) *Considerations for Working with People Who Self-Harm*. Information Sheet G12. Lutterworth: BACP.

Allen, C. (1995) 'Helping with deliberate self-harm: some practical guidelines'. *Journal of Mental Health* 4, pp. 243–50.

Chapter 8
Ethical issues

It is helpful to think of ethics as being relevant to our practice as counsellors at two levels: a means through which we can set parameters of good practice; and a way of thinking that is embedded in everything we do. I shall explain these two ideas in a little more detail. First, many counsellors think of ethics as outlining the key boundaries between what we should do, can do, and should not do in our work. We know, for example, that it is 'ethically wrong' to financially or sexually exploit our clients, and that we should not pretend to be able to offer something we are not qualified or experienced to deliver safely. We use ethics as a means of setting boundaries and distinctions between what is 'good' and what is 'bad'. While this is an important approach to ethics, it tends to be quite binary in nature, in that something is either okay, or not okay.

The second way of approaching ethics therefore, takes us beyond this binary, two-dimensional way of thinking and instead allows us to reflect more deeply on our work with a more dynamic, three-dimensional approach. I recently heard Tim Bond, author of BACP's *Ethical Framework for Good Practice in Counselling and Psychotherapy* (hereinafter referred to as the *Ethical Framework*: BACP, 2010) talk about this approach as an 'ethical engagement'. That is, as counsellors we engage with ethical thinking in a meaningful but ongoing way, rather than simply allowing ourselves to think about ethics as rule-setting. This second approach allows us perhaps to access the nuances of our work with clients more effectively.

This chapter will probably pay less attention to the first approach to ethics (the one I described as 'binary') and will instead reflect more on the second, which I will call a 'dimensional' approach. This is because I will make an assumption that as readers of this book you will be familiar with the 'rights' and 'wrongs' of counselling practice and, if not, other books exist that would provide a much better insight than I have space for here. I have made a couple of recommendations at the end of this chapter for further reading. Rather, when working with self-harm in a counselling relationship we need to reflect on dimensional ethics as a means of creating, maintaining and reviewing a safe and appropriate therapeutic space. To do this I will make reference to BACP's *Ethical Framework* as a means of helping us to negotiate a way through our thinking. I will use this document simply because as BACP is the UK's largest counselling and psychotherapy professional body it is likely that the majority of the readers of this book will be familiar with it. There are, of course, several other key ethically-orientated documents, including: UKCP's *Ethical Principles and Code of Professional Conduct* (UKCP, 2009); BABCP's *Standards of Conduct, Performance and Ethics in the Practice of Behavioural and Cognitive Psychotherapies* (BABCP, 2012); and the Counselling and Psychotherapy in Scotland's (COSCA) *Statement of Ethics and Code of Practice* (COSCA, 2011), for example.

The *Ethical Framework* outlines three key areas for consideration: values; principles; and personal moral qualities, before moving on to 'good practice' guidance. My intention is to take each of these initial areas in turn and explore its importance and application in our work with clients where self-harm is a feature.

Values

The *Ethical Framework* (p. 2) outlines key values of counselling and psychotherapy. I have slightly re-ordered them here from the way they appear in the original document. Here I have grouped them together into two key areas: **relational**, (to do with ourselves and the nature of the relationship); and societal, (to do with the wider nature of counselling and psychotherapy provision, its effectiveness and how it is contextualised at a societal level).

- Relational
    - Ensuring the integrity of practitioner-client relationships
    - Enhancing the quality of relationships between people
    - Protecting the safety of clients
    - Fostering a sense of self that is meaningful to the person(s) concerned
    - Increasing personal effectiveness
- Societal
    - Respecting human rights and dignity
    - Alleviating personal distress and suffering
    - Striving for the fair and adequate provision of counselling and psychotherapy services
    - Enhancing the quality of professional knowledge and its application
    - Appreciating the variety of human experience and culture

Relational

Relational values are to do with ourselves and the nature of the therapeutic relationship. They attend to important areas of both practice and 'being', (that is, our sense of ourselves and our client's sense of us). We can quickly see how values contribute to the dimensional nature of ethics, in that how we are in a therapeutic relationship is more than simply knowing what is 'right' and 'wrong', but also encompasses how we work at the integrity and quality of our relationships as well as privileging the meaningful experience of the client in a safe and respectful way.

Activity

Reflect on the following questions to do with relational values, with respect to yourself and your experience of being in relationships:
1 What are the most important aspects of personal relationships for you?
2 What are the most important aspects of therapeutic relationships for you?
3 What are the key similarities and differences between your personal and therapeutic relationships?
4 What actions do you take to ensure the integrity of your personal and therapeutic relationships?
5 What do the answers to the questions above mean for how you see yourself in the world?

Voices

Suky

Suky is a counsellor who works in a high-security male prison. Her client, Eddie, is a 20-year-old Afro-Caribbean man serving a sentence of four years for assault, carried out when he was 18. He is depressed and withdrawn and has been sent for counselling because of recurrent self-harm, cutting himself on his legs and arms. Suky sees him in her counselling room, which is adjacent to the block of cells in which Eddie lives. During sessions a prison warden stands outside the counselling room in case of potential violence. Eddie says he finds the sessions with Suky helpful but is reluctant to say too much because of the limited confidentiality Suky is able to offer.

Suky's work with Eddie raises a number of important issues that are based not only in binary ethics, but also dimensional ethics too. Suky has to work within a strict and limited contract of confidentiality and is very aware of her responsibilities towards Eddie both in her work and for his safety. However, Suky also has to attend to the dimensional ethics and how aspects of her working environment shape and influence the nature of the relationship. The influencing factors might include:

- Suky's sense of self in the context of a high-security setting
- Eddie's sense of self in the context of a high-security setting
- Suky's perception of Eddie as a violent man at high risk
- Eddie's perception of Suky as a female counsellor and her relational 'difference' in an otherwise all-male setting
- the limitations imposed on Eddie's autonomy and freedom of action
- **transferential** and **countertransferential** dynamics informed both by the relationship and the setting.

Let us focus specifically on Suky's perception of Eddie as a violent man at high risk. The environment in which Eddie lives defines him by his past behaviour and current actions: he is a violent man (because of the assault) and is high risk (because of his depression and self-harm). The values of counselling would define Eddie differently, focusing instead on the 'person' of Eddie and his potential for growth and change. Dimensional ethics requires Suky to reflect deeply on these areas to help her reconnect with Eddie's human-ness and his potential for growth, without responding to him as defined by the environment. In this instance the context defines the goals of counselling as a reduction in Eddie's self-harm (and thus the perceived risk), while Eddie's hopes for counselling might be very different. An important point therefore, is to be aware of the impact of external factors on the nature and form of the relationship, and how the needs of others' can prioritise self-harm as the point of change.

Societal

Societal values are those aspects that fall outside the immediacy of the therapeutic relationship but are instead contextualising factors that inform its nature. We might agree that counselling is about alleviating personal distress and suffering and respecting others' rights, but such values would also include the equitable provision of counselling (not discriminating on the basis of wealth, culture, age, disability, gender, sexuality, etc), the acknowledgement of difference and recognition of the importance of knowledge in the **process** of change.

Activity

Consider the following questions that are to do with how you position yourself in relation to societal values:

1 What are your personal 'benchmarks' for knowing whether your human rights are being respected by others?
2 What does 'dignity' mean to you?
3 How do you experience your position in society, with respect to: choice; freedom and autonomy; and knowledge?
4 As a counsellor how do you ensure your services are accessible to all those that need it, within your working context?
5 How do your gender, age, culture, sexuality and physical and intellectual abilities inform and shape your sense of self in society?

If we return to Suky and Eddie, we can immediately see how the values of counselling have the potential to be compromised by a number of factors, including:

- the societal stereotypes that permeate around the nature of being male, young and black
- fears associated with violence and unpredictability
- perceptions society holds about prisoners and their relative rights and influence
- debates around prison as a place for punishment or rehabilitation
- perceptions held by society about counselling either as a viable intervention or a 'soft option'.

Perceptions held by society about self-harm range from regarding it as an act of 'madness' or a strategy for coping. If we position ourselves at one point of a continuum in relation to the above considerations, we might wonder why Eddie should deserve counselling at all given his offending behaviour and his ongoing violent acts (albeit against himself). However, counselling would not take this position and, as a counsellor, Suky needs to find a way of negotiating her way through these perceptions, including her own stereotypes of people (because arguably we internalise perceptions as a consequence of growing up in a culture where such stereotypes abound). For Suky to work effectively with Eddie (whether or not that includes specifically with his self-harm), respecting his human rights and dignity and working towards his potential for growth, she needs to reflect carefully on how counselling values might be impinged or undermined.

Principles

The *Ethical Framework* (pp. 3–4) talks of the following principles that underpin counselling:

- being trustworthy, or demonstrating fidelity (honouring the trust placed in the practitioner)
- autonomy (respecting the client's autonomy)
- beneficence (promoting the client's well-being)
- non-maleficence (avoiding harm to the client)
- justice (fair and impartial treatment of all clients)
- self-respect (fostering self-knowledge and self-care).

We will consider the points above in relation to Suky and Eddie's counselling, and specifically around their potential work in response to Eddie's self-harm.

Being trustworthy/demonstrating fidelity

Arguably all counselling relationships require trust: trust in the client's **capacity** to change and engage in a **process** of change, and the client's capacity to trust the practitioner's willingness and ability to offer appropriate help. It might be that Eddie comes to counselling with a willingness to trust Suky from the outset, but equally there may be a number of factors that might impair his capacity to trust, such as his previous experiences of relationships (including familial ones), society's response to him (which might include racism and discrimination), and being in prison where his freedom and choices are limited. Unlike most other clients, Eddie has not had the choice whether or not to **disclose** his self-harm to his counsellor, instead this has been disclosed for him with a requirement for Suky to reduce his risk (presumably by reducing his self-harm). He might therefore be wary and suspicious of Suky as just another part of a system that, from his perspective, disempowers him and disregards his privacy and dignity.

The early stages of counselling will be important in helping Eddie begin to trust both Suky, and also counselling. Talking through how confidentiality will apply to their relationship, particularly in the context of the institution's perception of Eddie as being 'at risk' because of his self-harm, will help Eddie begin to understand the parameters of what he can share and, in doing so, help him begin to develop the early stages of trust. Suky communicating that counselling need not be about his self-harm if that is not his primary focus will help Eddie to feel that Suky might be more interested in what he has to say, rather than others' views. This is true in all working contexts where clients need to be able to trust the parameters of counselling, but also the integrity of their counsellor and their counsellor's capacity and willingness to hear their story.

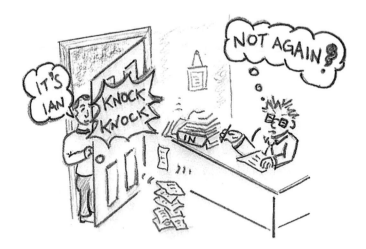

Figure 8.1 The counsellor's capacity to hear the client's story

Autonomy

Picking up from the last point above, trust will also grow from the client's perceived level of autonomy in the counselling relationship. This is particularly true when self-harm is a feature of a client's difficulties, in that it is often a difficulty for others, particularly friends and family. Like Eddie, clients will often be 'encouraged' to attend counselling when self-harm becomes apparent because of the anxieties of others and the hope that a counsellor will be able to 'sort it out'. The prison has anxieties about Eddie's self-harm, but in other situations it might be a parent, or a partner or friend.

It can be enormously liberating for clients for a counsellor to ask them whether it is their self-harm they wish to focus on, or instead something else. Just as Suky might explore with Eddie his motivations for counselling and the areas he might wish to discuss, rather than assuming self-harm must inevitably be the focus of attention.

Beneficence

Eddie's self-harm is of concern for those entrusted with his care. Likewise, knowing that someone close to us is harming themselves is likely to bring about strong feelings of wanting to 'make it better'. As a counsellor too, we might be drawn to act in such a way to help the client stop harming themselves believing that is the best way of promoting the client's well-being. As we know, however, from other aspects of work with clients, simply doing things in an attempt to help them feel better is not necessarily the same as beneficence. Promoting a client's well-being is much more about providing them with an appropriately confidential and respectful space in which they can explore difficulties and find workable solutions. Not all problems can be solved, so sometimes counselling is about finding better ways of managing difficulties.

Suky cannot deal with Eddie's immediate day-to-day predicament, in that he is serving a prison sentence and has to contend with the particular challenges of living in that environment. Instead, her task is about creating a space in counselling where Eddie can explore his concerns with dignity and respect, setting his own parameters and priorities. We cannot assume that promoting the client's well-being equates to sorting problems out for them.

Non-maleficence

Perhaps the principle of non-maleficence is one of the most challenging areas of practice for counsellors in working with clients where risk is an issue, whether it be suicidal potential or self-harm, by virtue of the fact that the client doing things that are harmful seems to go against the principle of non-maleficence. Obviously, our responsibility is to our clients, rather than for our clients. That is, we have a responsibility for the aspects of counselling that we have control over, but we cannot be responsible for all that our client does or says, either during counselling or outside of it.

Within a binary approach to ethical thinking we can be clear about the importance of not acting in a way that would cause a client harm. From a more dimensional perspective, however, when working with self-harm our actions need to be focused on the client's capacity to understand their self-harming actions, as well as supporting ways in which they might begin to find more self-caring ways of responding to their distress. Eddie cuts himself on his arms and legs, presumably in response to levels of distress he otherwise finds difficult to contain or express. Suky's responsibility is not to stop Eddie's self-harm (while that might be the priority of the institution), but rather to help Eddie explore the meaning of his self-harm so that he can begin to find his alternative strategies of coping. In doing so Suky would be mindful of not acting in a way that would cause harm, but rather to retain Eddie's dignity and integrity to help him in moving towards self-care.

Justice

Individual or institutional anxieties around self-harm can often lead to policies or actions that might compromise the principle of justice. People who self-harm who have attended A&E departments, for example, some-times have very negative experiences of how they are treated (Spandler, 2001). Such responses are not confined to medical settings; I have known of counselling services who have withdrawn counselling if clients are known to self-harm and will not reinstate it until they report they have stopped. This position is certainly informed by a 'them and us' philo-sophical view of self-harm, which I have challenged throughout this book, and it could be argued might not meet the principle of justice under the *Ethical Framework*.

We must be willing to ensure that we respond to clients openly, fairly and honestly in all our interactions. There could be a danger of Suky reacting more to the institution's anxieties about Eddie's self-harm and responding to him differently than she might with other clients, perhaps by changing the nature of the confidentiality she is able to offer, or not allowing sufficient time or space for Eddie to set his own goals for coun-selling, instead imposing different, externally defined, priorities.

Self-respect

We have talked in detail in Chapter 5 of the importance of self-care. All counselling demands we take an explicit and active approach to how we care for ourselves, and this is particularly true for self-harm. It is important that we take steps to educate and inform ourselves about the nature and meaning of self-harm, our own self-harming processes, and the impact on clients as well as the impact of self-harming narratives on our own sense of self-support and integrity.

As we have outlined throughout this chapter, in different ways Suky has to manage a number of competing demands in her work with Eddie, in terms of her values, the principles of counselling and, as we will move on to, personal moral qualities. Without doubt, the successful management of such demands can bring about profoundly important work for vulner-able people finding ways through their distress. However, managing these demands can also bring about costs, which we must pay careful attention to.

Personal moral qualities

The *Ethical Framework* (p. 4) outlines the following moral qualities that counsellors should possess to meet the demands of ethical practice:

- empathy: the ability to communicate understanding of another person's experience from that person's perspective
- sincerity: a personal commitment to consistency between what is professed and what is done
- integrity: commitment to being moral in dealings with others, personal straightforwardness, honesty and coherence
- resilience: the capacity to work with the client's concerns without being personally diminished
- respect: showing appropriate esteem to others and their understanding of themselves
- humility: the ability to assess accurately and acknowledge one's own strengths and weaknesses
- competence: the effective deployment of the skills and knowledge needed to do what is required
- fairness: the consistent application of appropriate criteria to inform decisions and actions
- wisdom: possession of sound judgement that informs practice
- courage: the capacity to act in spite of known fears, risks and uncertainty.

It is not my intention to discuss each of the above in turn as they are self-explanatory. Suffice to say the skills outlined in Chapter 3 are rendered meaningless unless the above qualities are in place. Whether it is possible to teach such personal moral qualities, whether we are born with them, or instead whether they develop in response to our experience of such qualities in others who influence us is difficult to determine. When applied to Suky in her work with Eddie, their importance becomes apparent in helping Eddie contend with the very real challenges in his life, the consequence of previous harmful experiences and relationships, as well as finding a way of understanding, expressing and thus moving through his distress so that future harm is minimised.

....

Summary

In this chapter I have tried to outline some of the important elements in working ethically with self-harm in counselling. Clearly the points made here apply to all counselling, all of the time. However, I have also demonstrated that self-harm sometimes brings with it unique challenges in maintaining an ethical position. I have termed the 'rights' and 'wrongs' approach to ethics as a binary approach, whereas ethics as applied to the moment-by-moment aspect of our work I have termed dimensional ethics. Both are important, but as counsellors we tend to associate binary thinking with ethics more than we do dimensional thinking, which has an equal imperative. A bringing together of the two can help us meet our clients where they are at, as opposed to where we would like them to be and, in doing so, maintain a position of self-respect and self-care as practitioners. This latter point is vital, as how can we facilitate a movement from harm to care in others if we are not able or willing to demonstrate it in ourselves?

Further reading

British Association for Counselling and Psychotherapy (2010) *Ethical Framework for Good Practice in Counselling and Psychotherapy.* Lutterworth: BACP.

Bond, T. (2009) *Standards and Ethics for Counselling in Action: Third Edition.* London: Sage.

Gabriel, L. & Casemore, R. (2009) *Relational Ethics in Practice: Narratives from Counselling and Psychotherapy.* London: Routledge.

Chapter 9
Research

There is extensive research into self-harm but, much like that into suicide, it tends to focus either on numbers or **demographics**. That is to say, how many people harm themselves and the types of groups of people who might self-harm more than others (according to age, gender, etc). This is interesting information and a more detailed overview of related research outcomes can be found on the web pages of the University of Oxford Centre for Suicide Research (which includes research into self-harm) which is an excellent resource. The link for this website can be found under *Further reading* at the end of this chapter. I considered some of the *how many* questions in the introduction to this book. As stated earlier, inevitably the research into numbers of people who self-harm is limited because of the following factors:

- Different research studies define self-harm differently, with some only including specific types of self-injury.
- Some researchers place self-harm within a **psychopathological** frame, while others broaden their perspective to include a wider range of people.
- Statistics usually only give an insight into those people who have made contact with helping services, typically A&E departments, for treatment.
- In all likelihood the overwhelming majority of self-harm does not come to the attention of such treatment centres and so overall numbers are, at best, **extrapolations** of baseline figures (estimates based on the numbers we know and how they might be generalisable across a wider population).

Likewise, the research into demographic groups (groupings of people based on identifying factors, such as age, gender, etc.) again often relies on extrapolated figures; however, such information can be helpful at a policy level. For example, if research tells us that self-harm is particularly prevalent in a young people population then intervention opportunities can be targeted at that group. Underpinning this whole picture, of course, is the philosophical assumption that there is a discrete group of people who self-harm, and the rest who do not. As I have discussed throughout this book, while this may be a help-ful position for **quantitative** analyses of raw data relating to numbers, particularly when applied to self-injury specifically, there is much to be gained, from a therapeutic perspective, from reflecting on our own self-harming behaviour, which might present in all sorts of ways (from drinking heavily when stressed, or driving recklessly when angry, for example).

For the purposes of this chapter I intend to offer an insight into some of the research that explores the *why* of self-harm, as opposed to the *how many* or *who*. This focus of research can be particularly helpful to us as counsellors in gaining an insight into the **processes** that might underpin self-harm. This can facilitate psychological contact with our clients and help provide a structure of thinking through which we can support cli-ents in their own increased self-understanding and thus, in time, to make changes from self-harm to self-care.

The limit of words means that it will not be possible to provide a com-plete coverage of all the research available. To look at specific aspects of self-harm relevant to your own setting or practice area it would be useful to undertake your own research, by accessing an academic re-search database, such as **PsychINFO** or, if you do not have access to such academic resources, such information is also available via Google Scholar (**http://scholar.google.co.uk**). Some papers are freely available online, while others require you to pay for them. A good overview of each paper should be freely available in every instance via the **abstract**, which will provide a summary of the focus of the paper and any key findings. This will help you to ensure you select papers only directly relevant to your area of interest.

I intend to highlight some interesting and relevant research across four key areas:

- **modality**-specific research
- influences of culture, gender and age
- particular therapeutic perceptions and strategies
- counsellor perspectives

Modality-specific research

Research has been undertaken into a number of different approaches to working with self-harm from a modality-specific perspective, (that is, from a particular theoretical orientation). Slee et al (2008) undertook a **randomised controlled trial** (RCT) looking at cognitive-behavioural (CBT) interventions. Participants, who were people already identified as self-harming and aged 15–35 years old, were randomly allocated to one of two groups: the treatment 'as usual' group (medication, general psychotherapy and hospitalisation), or a group who received CBT. The researchers found that those who were in the CBT group had 'significantly greater reductions in self-harm, suicidal cognitions and symptoms of depression and anxiety' (p. 202) and improvements in self-esteem and problem-solving abilities. Moorey (2010) again looked at CBT as an approach for working with self-harm and considered a range of interventions with the CBT paradigm, concluding that CBT 'may be an effective treatment for deliberate self-harm' (p. 142). Other evidence for approaches related to CBT includes problem-solving therapy (Gratz, 2006; Muehlenkamp, 2006), cognitive-analytic therapy (Bateman & Fonagy, 2001; Ryle, 2004) and dialectical behaviour therapy (DBT) (Linehan, 1993)

Further work on DBT came from Feigenbaum (2010), who looked at DBT as a treatment for self-harm, noting that self-harm, 'is a solution to the problem of overwhelming and painful affective states' (p. 129), rather than the problem itself. This is consistent with the perspective I have taken throughout this book. Feigenbaum goes on to state, 'DBT may offer a range of skills to provide individuals with a repertoire of emotional regulation strategies as an alternative to self-harming strategies' (p. 130).

Allied to, but discrete from, CBT, compassion-focused therapy (CFT) has several core components, including 'caring and concern for the well-being of others; empathy and sympathy … ; recognition and tolerance of another's pain, without judging that person's situation or behaviors; and emotional warmth' (van Vliet & Kalnins, 2011, p. 300). CFT draws on a range of techniques, including CBT, humanistic relational principles and mindfulness, for example. While van Vliet and Kalnins advocate CFT as an approach for working with self-harm, they do acknowledge it as an emerging therapeutic approach with the need for more outcome research.

Shame is an important aspect central to the theoretical and philosophical framework of CFT and, as we have discussed at various stages throughout the book, can also be central to a self-harming process. Gilbert et al (2010) considered the importance of shame, self-criticism and social rank (how high or low a person feels about themselves in relation to others). They noted in their results that feelings of inferiority and shame were associated with self-harm, with self-criticism particularly linked with self-harm, depression and anxiety. They conclude that, 'a focused approach on self-critical styles and their origins may provide new lines in research and a focus for therapeutic interventions' (p. 573); this may further indicate the value of CFT in this context.

Motz (2010), taking a more psychoanalytic position, considers the importance of early attachment experiences and the 'particular importance of the skin' (p. 81) in understanding self-harm later on, 'which serve to communicate distress, anger, protest and the hope that a real attempt will be made to relate to the person who self-harms' (p. 81). Motz concludes her paper with a positive statement about the potential efficacy of counselling for self-harm, and particularly its relational quality. This is affirmed in the work of Adshead (2010) who also believes self-harm to be a form of communication.

Finally, work has been undertaken in the humanistic field. Of particular note is the work of Inckle (2010), who has undertaken extensive work into holistic and creative responses to self-harm arguing they can, 'offer practitioners opportunities to build a broad repertoire of healing interventions and supports for their clients' (p. 160).

Influences of culture, gender and age

Backman (2011) offers a helpful overview of self-harm as it presents across western culture, and states that, 'non-suicidal self-injurious behavior occurs in almost all cultures in various contexts' (p. 4), linking self-harm to ritual healing, religion, making a political statement or affirmation of identity. This may be linked to Turp's (2003) concept of 'culturally acceptable self-harming activities' (CASHA) (p. 9), including the use of tobacco, alcohol, recreational drugs, body-contact sports, sleep deprivation, tattooing, body-piercing and over-work (p. 10). Backman additionally notes that, 'In other cultures, non-suicidal self-injury is accepted and understood within certain contexts' (p. 5). An important conclusion to Backman's paper is the need to approach self-harm from a position that takes into account cultural and societal influence and how such influence will shape both the nature of self-harm and how it is perceived. She states that, 'To do this, we must make ourselves aware of our own cultural biases that our society has imparted on us' (p. 9).

Latzman et al (2010) note the influence of culture and gender on self-harm. In their study looking at a particular population in a poor area of the United States, they noted the highest risk group was that of African-American boys. Level of academic achievement was also linked with levels of self-harm, with the authors highlighting the need for further research in this area. Brausch and Gutierrez (2010) looked at differences between suicide attempts and self-harm in a group of adolescents. They found that those adolescents who identified that their self-harm was about coping rather than dying demonstrated generalised lower suicidal ideation, greater self-esteem and better parental support. The implication of their study is a need for the careful assessment of suicide potential with people who self-harm and the importance of the counsellor in not making assumptions about suicide potential simply because self-harm is part of the person's struggle. They further state that, 'helping to bolster self-esteem and self-evaluations, as well as involving and strengthening the adolescent's relationship with parental figures, could be beneficial to at-risk adolescents and significantly decrease their risk for suicide' (p. 241).

Looking specifically at the needs of adolescents in a school environment, Best (2006) studied the nature of self-harming in school settings and identified behaviours ranging from cutting through to unnecessary risk-taking. Best suggests in his paper that teachers' understanding of self-harm is 'patchy' (p. 161) and that teacher reactions to the **disclosure** of self-harm include, 'shock, panic and anxiety' (p. 161).

An under-researched area is that of self-harm amongst older people (research typically focuses on young people and adolescents). Dennis and Owens (2012) argue for specialist assessment and care for older people and state that, 'Evidence suggests that non-fatal and fatal self-harm are more closely related in older than in younger adults' (p. 356).

Research also explores the particular needs of other groups, such as those with intellectual disabilities (Brown & Baeil, 2009) who state that self-harm amongst this group often occurs within an interpersonal context and that 'traumatic early experiences of loss and abuse hold meaning in relation to this area' (p. 512). There is also a need for research into self-harm in men, where Taylor (2003) states that self-harm 'is even less acknowledged, accepted and understood than it is in women' (p. 83).

Finally, we highlighted in earlier chapters possible triggers for self-harm. Fliege et al (2009) offer a **systematic review** of the evidence looking at particular risk factors, which is a helpful study to refer to in obtaining a broader view of risk factors and their associated evidence-base.

Particular therapeutic perceptions and strategies

Allen (1995) categorises the reasons for self-harm into three primary groups: to manage moods or feelings; as a response to beliefs or habitual thoughts; and to manage interactions with others (pp. 244–5). She raises a number of important considerations for working with self-harm, including (pp. 245–6):

- A diagnosis of borderline personality disorder is often made in response to self-harm. While there may be psychiatric validity in such a diagnosis, such a diagnosis is more likely if the psychiatrist finds the patient a nuisance or dislikes them (Lewis a& Appleby, 1988).
- It is important to keep in mind the range of psychological interventions with an evidence-base for working effectively with self-harm (see the previous section on **modality**-specific research).
- It is wrong (and potentially harmful) to assume that any kind of counselling, 'even from an untrained or inexperienced helper' (p. 246) is better than no counselling at all. It is important to ensure that both counselling and the setting in which it is delivered is carefully structured, contracted and goals agreed.
- Counsellors who work with self-harm should ensure a level of competency and training, with an awareness of the key issues around self-harm.

Walker (2009) highlights the importance of understanding the relation-ship between self-harm and a person's self-agency (their capacity to support themselves and to facilitate change). She highlights how the 'external signs of self-harm may take over their identity and how others communicate and interact with them' (p. 122). We have discussed this concept throughout the book: the importance of counsellors ensuring they remain focused on the wider needs of the client and the specific areas of difficulty outlined in their **narrative**, rather than becoming self-harm focused. Walker's research affirms this point strongly and flags the potential harm to the therapeutic relationship and process should the counsellor begin to form a relationship with the self-harm, rather than the person themselves.

This point is further supported by the work of Hill and Dallos (2011), who explored narratives around self-harm amongst adolescents. They noted that their participants 'perceive a severe lack of understanding from others about self-harm, which appeared to inhibit them from developing coherent narratives' (p. 1). In short, if we as counsellors do not come to the counselling relationship with some understanding, in general terms, of the process and experience of self-harm we run the risk of inhibiting our clients' understanding of their self-harm too. Hill and Dallos argue (pp. 14-15) that work with young people (and arguably anyone who brings an experience of self-harm to the counselling process) should:

- not simply focus on why self-harm is happening, but also explore underlying issues and dynamics
- help the client to integrate previous traumatic or distressing life events into their wider 'life story' (p. 15)
- be cautious about medicalising an understanding about self-harm (such as a diagnosis of borderline personality disorder) as the relational and emotional struggles may easily be obscured by it
- work carefully with anger, so that clients are facilitated to find safe ways of expressing their anger, rather than further internalising it and thus creating more energy for their self-harm
- ensure there is space and time to facilitate a discussion of important previous experiences and help the client find ways of verbalising their experiences.

This latter point is particularly true when working with clients who struggle to find an emotional language for their experience. This is sometimes termed as 'alexithymia', and while such terminology is not necessary to help a client, knowing such terms can facilitate further research and reading. For example, Levant (1998) coined the term 'normative male alexithymia' to describe the difficulty of many males to articulate emotional content in their day-to-day narrative and experience (Englar-Carlson, 2006). Certainly in counselling, men will often struggle to meet the 'emotional benchmark' counsellors will often set for them and can find therapy a difficult and challenging process. This has implications for working with men who self-harm in that we may need to work differently to ensure men can use their own language to express difficulty or hurt, which might otherwise be articulated through a self-harming process.

Finally, the use of 'no-harm' contracts (where the counsellor contracts with a client not to harm themselves during the course of counselling or between sessions) is considered by Hyldahl and Richardson (2011). Often used in approaches such as DBT (Linehan, 1993), Hyldahl and Richardson identify a number of positive and negative aspects of such contracts and make a number of recommendations (pp. 124–6), including:

- any such contract is only as good as the relationship in which it is based
- the counsellor should always respect the autonomy of the client and any such contract should be collaborative
- avoid the use of the term 'contract'; instead using terms such as 'agreement'
- therapeutic focus should always be on the client's capacity for self-care and thinking differently about themselves, rather than simply agreeing to avoid a particular form of behaviour
- a client's struggle to hold to any agreement, or to refuse such an agreement, should be viewed as important feedback on the therapeutic relationship; such agreements form only part of any management of risk.

There is not a great deal of research to demonstrate a sound evidence-base for the use of such contracts (Walsh, 2006). I would also personally concur with Simon (1999, p. 449) who suggests that those counsellors who believe such contracts demonstrate effective response to risk should keep in mind that using them 'merely creates an illusion of safety when it is not combined with competent treatment and management'. In short, it is always preferable to work collaboratively and relationally with a client around their self-harm rather than fall back on a contract or agreement that has the potential, at best, to be benign in its meaninglessness or, at worst, malignant should a client feel they have let their counsellor down by failing to adhere to it.

Counsellor perspectives

It is important to consider counsellor perspectives when working with self-harm. I have flagged throughout the book the importance of counsellors reflecting on their own attitudes towards and biases against self-harm and those factors that might facilitate but also impair true psychological connection with a client.

Fox (2011), following a **qualitative** study with a group of counsellors, found that for her participants working with self-harm raised a number of important challenges, including how best to work under organisational policy; the emotional impact of such work on the counsellor; the expectations of reducing or stopping self-harm and the role of supervision in supporting practice.

Long and Jenkins (2010), following their qualitative study with counsellors, affirmed the importance of the therapeutic relationship in working with self-harm because of the importance of 'time, confidentiality, acceptance, equality and sensitivity' (p. 196). Additionally, in terms of the process of the relationship the researchers identified the importance of 'hope, trust, presence; openness; "*being new*" with the client' (p. 197). They conclude that, 'All counsellors who encounter self-harm in their professional and personal lives have a pivotal role to play in improving the lives of people who self-harm. Counsellors' insight to the breadth and depth of self-harm behaviour can foster understanding and acceptance, while also challenging negative attitudes' (p. 199).

Turp (1999) affirms the importance of counsellor self-care when working with self-harm, as we have identified at various stages through this book, when she states, 'the price of regaining a feeling of aliveness and reality is very high, in terms of the negative experiences, both internal and external, which follow in the wake of self-harm' (p. 317). This is particularly true in the context of the findings by Fleet and Mintz (2012) who note that counsellors can experience a range of feelings in response to their client's self-harm, including 'shock; sadness; anxiety; anger; and frustration' (p. 1). They conclude by stressing the importance of self-care given the emotional and psychological impact of such work, and the need for more research into this area.

Finally, in considering the attitudes of clients who self-harm towards services that offer treatment and support, Taylor et al (2009) note that clients identified the need for improvement in how assessments were undertaken, as well as the choices available for support. They cited poor communication and a perceived lack of staff knowledge as being exacerbating factors. These have important implications for counsellors in their working with self-harm with clients, in the importance of communicating clearly about the place and meaning of counselling, carefully assessing the needs of client's as well as their particular hopes and goals for their work, and being informed about practice.

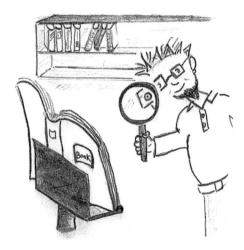

Figure 9.1 Research

Summary

There is extensive research into self-harm, much of which, however, attends to the *how much* and *who* questions. In this chapter we have highlighted some of the interesting literature that explores the *why* of self-harm and ways of working more effectively with it. A dominant theme is the importance of counsellors having an understanding of the nature and process of self-harm, communicating clearly with clients, focusing on the relational aspects of the client's experience, as well as helping clients to find meaning and expression for themselves. Underpinning this is the need for counsellors to ensure they pay careful attention to self-care.

Further reading

University of Oxford Centre for Suicide Research (including self-harm). **http://cebmh.warne.ox.ac.uk/csr/**

Multi-centre Study of Self-Harm in England. **http://cebmh.warne.ox.ac. uk/csr/mcm/**

Glossary

Abstract
A short piece of writing, usually at the beginning of an academic document, providing a summary of the contents.

Bibliotherapy
The provision of self-help support through the use of printed material, such as websites, books, self-help leaflets, etc.

Capacity
This is both a legal term (under the Mental Capacity Act 2005 or, in Scotland, the Adults with Incapacity Act (Scotland) 2000) which describes a person's ability to make informed decisions for themselves. If used in a therapeutic context, it will refer to the counsellor or client's ability to cope with or manage something within the therapeutic context (for example, the client's capacity to explore emotional material).

Congruence
A term primarily used in humanistic counselling. Refers to the counsellor's willingness and ability to share with the client their experience of the client's process and aspects of the therapeutic relationship.

Countertransference/countertransferential
A term mainly used in psychodynamic or psychoanalytic therapy, it also has relevance for other approaches too. Refers to a counsellor's response to a client that might be informed by other factors beyond the immediacy of the therapeutic relationship.

Demographic
A group with particular characteristics, (for example, based on age, gender, culture, etc.).

Disclosure
A willingness to share something personal about self, either in relation to the client or the counsellor (self-disclosure).

Dissociate
A psychological defence mechanism where the person unconsciously disconnects from strong, distressing or overwhelming feelings.

Early Intervention Team
A team of workers, usually based in a mental health setting, with a specific remit to offer immediate support to young people experiencing a first episode of psychosis.

Extrapolate/extrapolations
To infer or estimate from a specific set of data to a wider group or phenomenon.

Habitual
A recurring pattern of behaviour, thinking or feeling without conscious or deliberate intention.

Identification
Where a counsellor or client recognises an aspect of the other's experience in themselves.

Intrapersonal
The experience of a relationship with self; an internal process.

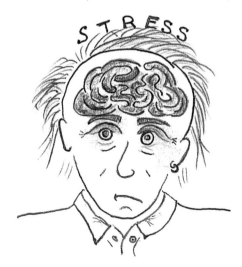

Figure 10.1 Intrapersonal

Interpersonal
The experience of a relationship with another; an external process.

Macro
Considering something from a bigger perspective, taking lots of information into account.

Meta
Meta can mean different things depending on the context. In terms of meta-narrative, as I have used it in this text, I mean a client's story or experience that brings together a number of aspects of what they do or say in therapy. In research terms, meta (as in meta-analysis) develops perspectives and conclusions integrated from a number of different sources.

Micro
Considering something from a specific or particular perspective; taking only one aspect of information into account.

Modality
In counselling terms, a particular model of training (such as person-centred, cognitive-behavioural therapy).

Munchausen's disorder
A diagnostic term used to describe a person who seeks out medical attention for themselves for health problems that are imagined.

Narrative
A story, or an account of an experience(s).

Process
In counselling terms, the ongoing features of a relationship that can contribute to awareness and change.

PsychINFO
A searchable academic database containing records of published research papers.

Psychopathological
A way of thinking or being that might relate to a diagnosable mental disorder or dysfunction.

Psychosis
A diagnostic term used to describe chaotic, disordered or disturbed thinking, sometimes accompanied by visual or auditory hallucinations.

Randomised controlled trial (RCT)
An approach to research, which typically makes use of large groups of people randomly assigned to particular groups so that a specific hypothesis or treatment can be tested.

Relational
In counselling terms, the process by which counsellor and client interact; in relationship.

Qualitative
An approach to research that focuses on words and narrative as a means of gaining insight into a particular phenomenon.

Quantitative
An approach to research that makes use of statistical analysis of numbers to generate transferable knowledge.

Safeguarding
The term used to describe a set of expectations, policies and procedures used to promote the well-being of children and young people, which would include child protection.

Statutory
Where an act or responsibility is defined in law; or where an organisation is funded centrally to fulfil a specific function(s), for example, Social Care Departments.

Systematic review
An approach to research where a number of research studies are evaluated against set criteria to obtain an overview of understanding of knowledge.

Systemic
A way of thinking about the systems in which people live and function, (such as family, school, work).

Transference/transferential
A term usually used in psychodynamic or psychoanalytic therapy, but with relevance for other modalities. Describes the process by which a person relates to another drawing on unconscious experiences or memories that relate to another person or people.

World-view
A culturally informed position of seeing the world (for example, individualistic or community).

References

Adshead, G. (2010) 'Written on the body: Deliberate self-harm as a communication'. *Psychoanalytic Psychotherapy* 24 (2), pp. 69–80.

Allen, C. (1995) 'Helping with deliberate self-harm: Some practical guidelines'. *Journal of Mental Health* 4, pp. 243–50.

Babiker, G. & Arnold, L. (1997) *The Language of Injury: Comprehending Self-Mutilation.* Oxford: Wiley-Blackwell.

Backman, A. (2011) 'A critical analysis of non-suicidal self-injury in Western culture'. *Encephalon: The Pitzer College Student Journal of Psychology* 1 (Fall 2011), pp. 4–10.

Bateman, A. & Fonagy, P. (2001) 'Treatment of borderline personality disorder with psychoanalytically-orientated partial hospitalisation: An 18-month follow-up'. *American Journal of Psychiatry* 158, pp. 36–42.

Best, R. (2006) 'Deliberate self-harm in adolescence: A challenge for schools'. *British Journal of Guidance and Counselling* 34 (2), pp. 161–75.

Bond, T. (2009) *Standards and Ethics for Counselling in Action: Third Edition.* London: Sage.

Brausch, A. M. & Gutierrez, P. M. (2010) 'Differences in non-suicidal self-injury and suicide attempts in adolescents'. *Journal of Youth and Adolescence* 39, pp. 233–42.

British Association for Behavioural and Cognitive Psychotherapies (2012) *Standards of Conduct, Performance and Ethics in the Practice of Behavioural and Cognitive Psychotherapies.* Bury: BABCP. **www.babcp.com/ Files/About/conduct--ethics.pdf** (accessed 15 December 2012).

British Association for Counselling and Psychotherapy (2010) *Ethical Framework for Good Practice in Counselling and Psychotherapy.* Lutterworth: BACP.

Brown, J. & Beail, N. (2009) 'Self-harm among people with intellectual disabilities living in secure service provision: A qualitative exploration'. *Journal of Applied Research in Intellectual Disabilities* 22, pp. 503–13.

Counselling and Psychotherapy in Scotland (2011) *COSCA Statement of Ethics and Code of Practice.* Stirling: COSCA. **www.cosca.org.uk/ new_documents.php?headingno=2&heading=Ethics** (accessed 15 December 2012).

Dennis, M. S. & Owens, D. W. (2012) 'Self-harm in older people: A clear need for specialist assessment and care'. *The British Journal of Psychiatry* 200, pp. 356–58.

Englar-Carlson, M. (2006) 'Masculine norms and the therapy process', in M. Englar-Carlson & M. A. Stevens (eds) *In the Room with Men.* Washington DC: American Psychological Association.

Favazza, A. R. (1989) 'Why patients mutilate themselves'. *Hospital and Community Psychiatry* 40 (2), pp. 137–45.

Feigenbaum, J. (2010) 'Self-harm – the solution not the problem: The Dialectical Behaviour Therapy Model'. *Psychoanalytic Psychotherapy* 24 (2), pp. 115–34.

Fellman, J.D., Getis, A. & Getis, J. (2007) *Human Geography: Landscapes of Human Activities.* Maidenhead: McGraw-Hill.

Figley, C.R. (1995). 'Compassion fatigue as secondary traumatic stress disorder: An overview', in C.R. Figley (ed.) *Compassion fatigue: Coping with secondary stress disorder in those who treat the traumatised.* New York: Brunner/Mazel.

Fleet, D. & Mintz, R. (2012) 'Counsellors' perceptions of client progression when working with clients who intentionally self-harm and the impact such work has on the therapist'. *Counselling and Psychotherapy Research.* **www.tandfonline.com/doi/abs/10.1080/14733145.2012.69 8421** pp. 1–9.

Fliege, H., Lee, J-R., Grimm, A. & Klapp, B. F. (2009) 'Risk factors and correlates of deliberate self-harm behavior: A systematic review'. *Journal of Psychosomatic Research* 66, pp. 477–93.

Fox, C. (2011) 'Working with clients who engage in self-harming behaviour: Experiences of a group of counsellors'. *British Journal of Guidance and Counselling* 39 (1), pp. 41–51.

Gabriel, L. & Casemore, R. (2009) *Relational Ethics in Practice: Narratives from Counselling and Psychotherapy.* London: Routledge.

Gilbert, P., McEwan, K., Irons, C., Bhundia, R., Christie, R., Broomhead, C. & Rockliff, H. (2010) 'Self-harm in a mixed clinical population: The roles of self-criticism, shame and social rank'. *British Journal of Clinical Psychology* 49, pp. 563–76.

Gratz, K. L. (2006) 'Risk factors for deliberate self-harm among female college students: The role and interaction of childhood maltreatment, emotional inexpressivity, and affect intensity/reactivity'. *American Journal of Orthopsychiatry* 76, pp. 238–50.

Hawton, K., Zahl, D. & Weatherall, R. (2003) 'Suicide following deliberate self-harm: long-term follow-up of patients who presented to a general hospital'. *British Journal of Psychiatry* 182, pp. 537–42.

Hill, K. & Dallos, R. (2011) 'Young people's stories of self-harm: A narrative study'. *Clinical Child Psychology and Psychiatry* 17 (3), pp. 1–17.

Horrocks, J., House, A. & Owens, D. (2002) *Attendances in the accident and emergency department following self-harm; a descriptive study.* University of Leeds, Academic Unit of Psychiatry and Behavioural Sciences. **www.leeds.ac.uk/lihs/psychiatry/reports/selfharm_attendances_report.pdf**

Hyldahl, R. S. & Richardson, B. (2011) 'Key considerations for using no-harm contracts with clients who self-injure'. *Journal of Counselling and Development* 89, pp. 121–27.

Inckle, K (2010) 'At the cutting edge: creative and holistic responses to self-injury'. *Creative Nursing* 16 (4), pp. 160–66.

Inskipp, F. & Proctor, B. (1993) *Making the Most of Supervision.* Twickenham: Cascade.

Kapur, N., House, A. & Creed, F. et al (1998) 'Management of deliberate self-poisoning in adults in four teaching hospitals: descriptive study'. *British Medical Journal* (316), pp. 831–32.

Khele, S., Symons, C. & Wheeler, S. (2008) 'An analysis of complaints to the British Association for Counselling and Psychotherapy, 1996–2006'. *Counselling and Psychotherapy Research* 8 (2), pp. 124–32.

Larcombe, A. (2008) 'Self-Care', in W. Dryden & A. Reeves (eds) *Key Issues for Counselling in Action: Second Edition*. London: Sage, pp. 283–97.

Latzman, R. D., Gratz, K. L., Young, J., Heiden, L. J., Damon, J. D. & Hight, T. L. (2010) 'Self-injurious thoughts and behaviors among young in an underserved area of the Southern United States: Exploring the moderating roles of gender, racial/ethnic background, and school-level'. *Journal of Youth and Adolescence* 39, pp. 270–80.

Levant, R. F. (1998) 'Desperately seeking language: Understanding, assessing and treating normative male alexithymia', in W. S. Pollock and R. F. Levant (eds) *New Psychotherapy for Men*. New York: Wiley, pp. 35–56.

Lewis, G. & Appleby, L. (1988) 'Personality disorder: the patients psychiatrists dislike'. *British Journal of Psychiatry* 153, pp. 44–9.

Linehan, M. M. (1993) *Skills Training Manual for Treating Borderline Personality Disorder*. New York: Guildford.

Long, M. & Jenkins, M. (2010) 'Counsellors' perspectives on self-harm and the role of the therapeutic relationship for working with clients who self-harm'. *Counselling and Psychotherapy Research* 10 (3), pp. 192–200.

McLeod, J. (2010) 'The effectiveness of workplace counselling: a systematic review', *Counselling and Psychotherapy Research* 10 (4), pp. 238–48.

Melzer, H., Lader, D., Corbin, T., Singleton, N., Jenkins, R., & Brugha, T. (2002) *Non-fatal suicidal behaviour among adults aged 16 to 74 in Great Britain*. London: The Stationery Office.

Mental Health Foundation (2006) The Truth About Self-Harm: For Young People and their Friends and Families. London: Mental Health Foundation.

Moorey, S. (2010) 'Managing the unmanageable: Cognitive behaviour therapy for deliberate self-harm'. *Psychoanalytic Psychotherapy* 24 (2), pp. 135–49.

Motz, A. (2010) 'Self-harm as a sign of hope'. *Psychoanalytic Psychotherapy* 24 (2), pp. 81–92.

Muehlenkamp, J. J. (2006) 'Empirically supported treatments and general therapy guidelines for non-suicidal self-injury'. *Journal of Mental Health Counseling* 28, pp. 166–85.

National Institute for Health and Clinical Excellence (2004) *Self-harm: The short-term physical and psychological management and secondary prevention of self-harm in primary and secondary care (NICE Clinical Guidance 16)*. London: NICE.

National Institute for Health and Clinical Excellence (2011) *Self-Harm: Longer-term Management (NICE Clinical Guidance 133)*. Manchester: NICE.

National Self-Harm Network (1998) *Self-injury: myths and common sense.* National Self-Harm Network. **www.nshn.co.uk/facts.html**

Oxford Dictionaries Online, **www.oxforddictionaries.com**, accessed 28 February 2013.

Owens, D., Horrocks, J. & House, A. (2002) 'Fatal and non-fatal repetition of self-harm. Systematic review'. *British Journal of Psychiatry* 181, pp. 193–9.

Pearlman, L.A., & Saakvitne, K.W. (1995). Trauma and the therapist: Countertransference and vicarious traumatisation in psychotherapy with incest survivors. New York: W.W. Norton.

Pembroke, L.R. (ed) (1996) *Self-harm: Perspectives from Personal Experience*. London: Survivors Speak Out.

Reeves, A. (2010) *Counselling Suicidal Clients.* London: Sage.

Reeves, A. (2012) 'Working with suicide and self-harm in counselling', in C Feltham and I Horton (eds) *The SAGE Handbook of Counselling and Psychotherapy*. London: Sage, pp. 539–33.

Reeves, A. (2013) *An Introduction to Counselling and Psychotherapy: From Theory to Practice.* London: Sage.

Reeves, A. & Howdin, J. (2010) *Considerations for Working with People Who Self-Harm (Information Sheet G12).* Lutterworth: BACP.

Reeves, A. & Mintz, R. (2001) 'Counsellors' experiences of working with suicidal clients: an exploratory study', *Counselling and Psychotherapy Research* 1 (3), pp. 172–6.

Royal College of Psychiatrists (2010) *Self-Harm, Suicide and Risk: Helping People Who Self-Harm.* London: Royal College of Psychiatrists College Report CR158.

Royal College of Psychiatrists (2013) *Alternatives to Self-Harm and Distraction Techniques.* **www.rcpsych.ac.uk/PDF/Self-Harm Distractions and Alternatives FINAL.pdf** (accessed 17 December 2012).

Ryle, A. (2004) 'The contribution of cognitive analytic therapy to the treatment of borderline personality disorder'. *Journal of Personality Disorders* 18, pp. 3–35.

Sanderson, C. (2006) *Counselling Adult Survivors of Child Sexual Abuse (Third Edition).* London: Jessica Kingsley Publishers.

Schneidman, E. S. (1996) *The Suicidal Mind.* Oxford: Oxford University Press.

Sexton, L. (1999) 'Vicarious traumatisation of counsellors and effects on their workplaces'. *British Journal of Guidance & Counselling* 27 (3), pp. 393–403.

Simon, R. I. (1999) 'The suicide prevention contract: clinical, legal and risk management issues'. *Bulletin of the American Academy of Psychiatry and the Law* 27, pp. 445–50.

Slee, N., Garnefski, N., van der Leeded, R., Arensman, E. & Spivhoven, P. (2008) 'Cognitive-behavioural intervention for self-harm: randomised controlled trial'. *The British Journal of Psychiatry* 192, pp. 202–11.

Spandler, H. (2001) *Who's Hurting Who: Young People, Self-Harm and Suicide.* Gloucester: Handsell Publishing.

Symons, C. (2012) Complaints and Complaining in Counselling and Psychotherapy: Organisational and Client Perspectives. University of Leicester: Unpublished PhD Thesis.

Symons, C., Khele, S., Rogers, J., Turner, J. & Wheeler, S. (2011) 'Allegations of serious professional misconduct: an analysis of the British Association for Counselling and Psychotherapy's Article 4.6 cases, 1998–2007', *Counselling and Psychotherapy Research* 11 (4), pp. 257–65.

Taylor, B. (2003) 'Exploring the perspectives of men who self-harm'. *Learning in Health and Social Care* 2 (2), pp. 83–91.

Taylor, L. T., Hawton, K., Fortune, S. & Kapur, N. (2009) 'Attitudes towards clinical services among people who self-harm: systematic review'. *The British Journal of Psychiatry* 194, pp. 104–10.

Turp, M. (1999) 'Encountering self-harm in psychotherapy and counselling practice'. *British Journal of Psychotherapy* 15 (3), pp. 306–21.

Turp, M. (2003) *Hidden Self-Harm. Narratives from Psychotherapy.* London: Jessica Kingsley.

United Kingdom Council for Psychotherapy (2009) *Ethical Principles and Code of Professional Conduct.* London: UKCP. **www.psychotherapy.org. uk/code_of_ethics.html** (accessed 15 December 2012).

Van Vliet, K. J. & Kalnins, G. R. C. (2011) 'A compassion-focussed approach to non-suicidal self-injury'. *Journal of Mental Health Counseling* 33 (4), pp. 295–311.

Vicarious Trauma Institute (2012) *What is Vicarious Trauma?* **www. vicarioustrauma.com/whatis.html** (accessed 25 October 2012).

Walker, T. (2009) '"Seeing beyond the battled body" – An insight into self-hood and identity from women's accounts who self-harm with a diagnosis of borderline personality disorder'. *Counselling and Psychotherapy Research* 9 (2), pp. 122–8.

Walsh, B. W. (2006) *Treating Self-injury: A Practical Guide*. New York: Guildford Press.

Winter, D., Bradshaw, S., Bunn, F. & Wellsted, D. (2012a) 'A systematic review of the literature on counselling and psychotherapy for the prevention of suicide: 1. Quantitative outcome and process studies'. *Counselling and Psychotherapy Research*. iFirst.

Winter, D., Bradshaw, S., Bunn, F. & Wellsted, D. (2012b) 'A systematic review of the literature on counselling and psychotherapy for the prevention of suicide: 2. Qualitative Studies. *Counselling and Psychotherapy Research*. iFirst.

Index